YOUR COMPLETE GUIDE TO ALLERGIC RHINITIS

Learn How to Boost Your Immune System for Fighting Allergies, Hay Fever and Other Related Conditions with Over 100 Allergy-Friendly Recipes

Joe Miller, RD

COPYRIGHT PAGE

Table of Contents

INTRODUCTION

Rhinitis, characterized by inflammation of the nasal lining, manifests clinically through symptoms such as a runny nose, itching, sneezing, and nasal obstruction (congestion). It can be triggered by allergies, which may be seasonal (known as 'hay fever') or perennial, with common allergens including house dust mites, pets like cats and dogs, and molds. Infections also contribute to rhinitis, which can be either acute or persistent. Notably, rhinitis, whether allergic or not, serves as a risk factor for developing asthma and is associated with conditions like otitis media with effusion and sinusitis, often termed rhinosinusitis due to the involvement of the nasal passages.

Allergic rhinitis, affecting one in every four individuals in the United Kingdom, is prevalent, and its incidence is rising globally, particularly in Westernized societies. Despite its prevalence, allergic rhinitis is often overlooked or misattributed to recurring colds, especially in children, by family members, clinicians, and even patients themselves. However, disregarding allergic rhinitis is a significant oversight, as it not only diminishes quality of life but can also disrupt sleep, impair school performance, and affect work attendance. Moreover, allergic children are prone to more illnesses and face exacerbated issues with infections. For instance, asthmatic children with allergies, when exposed to high levels of triggering allergens, are significantly more likely to require hospitalization due to asthma exacerbation after catching a cold. Effective management of underlying allergic conditions can mitigate these challenges.

Additionally, allergic rhinitis might serve as an initial indication of broader allergic conditions, such as hay fever in adolescents or adults. If left untreated, rhinitis can progress to chronic symptoms characterized by nasal congestion, which can impact adjacent tissues including the sinuses, throat, middle ear, and bronchial tubes. Such cases necessitate further evaluation and treatment by an otolaryngologist or allergy specialist.

In summary, rhinitis, particularly allergic rhinitis, presents significant health implications beyond mere nasal symptoms. Recognizing and appropriately addressing this condition is crucial for improving overall well-being and mitigating the risk of complications associated with allergic diseases.

CHAPTER 1
ESSENTIAL INFORMATION
REGARDING ALLERGIC RHINITIS

Allergic rhinitis, medically termed as nasal lining irritation due to allergic stimuli, is a widespread condition often referred to as hay fever. Its prevalence is significant, impacting approximately 10-15% of children and 26% of adults in the United Kingdom alone, as of 2017. However, its influence extends far beyond mere statistics, as it adversely affects various aspects of life including quality of life, job performance, school attendance, and even poses a risk factor for the development of asthma. Over the past two decades, there has been a concerning threefold increase in the incidence of allergic rhinitis, highlighting its growing significance in public health discourse.

This condition, characterized by symptoms such as a runny nose, sneezing, and watery eyes, is primarily triggered by seasonal allergens like plant pollen. However, it can also manifest in response to non-seasonal allergens such as animal fur and dust. The terms hay fever and allergic rhinitis are often used interchangeably in medical discourse, reflecting their shared characteristics and symptoms.

In New Zealand, approximately 20% of the population experiences allergic rhinitis or hay fever, with onset often occurring in childhood, affecting about one-third of those affected before the age of ten. The impact of allergic rhinitis extends beyond the nasal passages, affecting the eyes, throat, and ears. Treatment typically involves a combination of allergen avoidance, medication, and immunotherapy to manage symptoms and prevent complications that could damage various parts of the respiratory system, sinuses, and middle ear.

Allergic rhinitis is predominantly mediated by immunoglobulin E (IgE), which interacts with allergens in the air, triggering mast cells to release inflammatory substances. These substances lead to typical symptoms such as nasal congestion, sneezing, and irritation, while also contributing to extranasal symptoms like allergic conjunctivitis and asthma. Despite affecting over 400 million individuals worldwide, allergic rhinitis remains often misdiagnosed and undertreated, adding to its burden on healthcare systems globally.

Moreover, the economic impact of allergic rhinitis is substantial, with direct medical expenditures reaching billions of dollars annually in the United States alone. The associated productivity losses further exacerbate the economic burden, surpassing that of several other chronic conditions combined. In countries with emerging economies, indirect losses impose additional challenges, further underlining the significant and often underestimated expense of allergic rhinitis.

Rhinitis, whether allergic or non-allergic, underscores the importance of understanding its diverse triggers and manifestations. While allergic rhinitis involves immune-mediated responses to various allergens, non-allergic rhinitis can result from factors like environmental pollutants, strong odors, or anatomical abnormalities. Proper management requires a comprehensive approach tailored to individual patient needs, emphasizing the importance of seeking timely medical attention and exploring effective treatment options to mitigate symptoms and improve overall quality of life.

Symptoms and Signs of Allergic Rhinitis

• Nasal congestion resulting from the swelling of the nasal mucous membranes.

• Sneezing, a runny nose, and watery eyes are common symptoms.

• Itchy sensations in the eyes, nose, roof of the mouth, or throat.

• Puffiness under the eyes and the appearance of dark circles.

• Snoring and coughing may also occur.

• Facial tension can contribute to discomfort.

Allergic rhinitis manifests whenever allergens are present, necessitating personalized solutions for each individual affected. However, the encouraging news is that with appropriate treatment and precautions, the unpleasant symptoms of allergic rhinitis can be alleviated or eliminated. This is particularly heartening for individuals with asthma, as hay fever is prevalent among asthmatics and can exacerbate asthma symptoms. Furthermore, early intervention holds promise in potentially preventing children with hay fever from developing asthma later in life.

Moreover, the impact of allergic rhinitis extends beyond physical discomfort, often affecting daily activities and overall quality of life. Individuals experiencing persistent symptoms may find themselves struggling to concentrate at work or school due to the constant distraction caused by nasal congestion, sneezing fits, and itchy eyes. Furthermore, the sleep disturbances caused by snoring and coughing can lead to fatigue and irritability during the day, compounding the challenges faced by those with allergic rhinitis.

Finding effective treatment options often involves a trial-and-error approach, as what works for one person may not necessarily work for another. However, advancements in medical research and treatment modalities offer hope for improved symptom management and better quality of life for individuals with allergic rhinitis. From over-the-counter antihistamines and nasal sprays to allergen immunotherapy, there are various avenues to explore under the guidance of healthcare professionals.

In addition to medical interventions, lifestyle modifications and environmental precautions can also play a significant role in minimizing exposure to allergens and reducing symptom severity. Strategies such as using allergen-proof bedding, keeping windows closed during peak pollen seasons, and regularly cleaning indoor spaces can help create a more allergen-free environment. Additionally, practicing good nasal hygiene, such as rinsing the nasal passages with saline solution, can help alleviate congestion and promote better breathing.

Furthermore, fostering awareness and understanding of allergic rhinitis within the community and among healthcare providers is essential for early detection and timely intervention. By promoting education and advocacy initiatives, we can empower individuals with allergic rhinitis to proactively manage their condition and seek the support they need to live well despite its challenges. Ultimately, by working together to address the multifaceted aspects of allergic rhinitis, we can strive towards a future where everyone affected by this condition can enjoy optimal health and well-being.

CHAPTER 2
WHAT LEADS TO ALLERGIC RHINITIS?

Allergic rhinitis, commonly referred to as hay fever, arises when the immune system reacts excessively to non-infectious particles like plant pollens, molds, dust mites, animal proteins, chemicals, foods, medications, insect venom, and various other triggers. During an allergic reaction, a specific antibody known as IgE binds to cells in the lungs, skin, and mucous linings of the body, prompting the release of histamine and other substances. These substances induce skin redness and swollen membranes by dilating blood vessels. When this reaction occurs in the nose, it leads to symptoms such as sneezing, itching, a runny nose, and congestion.

Seasonal allergic rhinitis is primarily triggered by certain plants that pollinate during specific seasons. For example, springtime allergies result from pollen from blooming trees, while grass pollination causes allergic reactions in early summer. Ragweed hypersensitivity is prevalent in the autumn, exacerbated by mold spores found on falling leaves during the fall season.

On the other hand, perennial allergic rhinitis can be caused by sensitivities to animal proteins, mold, houseplants, and dust mites commonly found in carpets and upholstery. When seeking medical attention for suspected allergic rhinitis, understanding the pattern of symptoms, including seasonal triggers, indoor versus outdoor exposure, specific triggers, and animal exposure, is crucial for accurate diagnosis and effective treatment.

Non-allergic rhinitis and vasomotor rhinitis, a subtype of non-allergic rhinitis, do not involve an allergic reaction and do not require the presence of IgE antibodies. Even individuals who test positive for allergies may experience non-allergic rhinitis. This type of rhinitis can be triggered by various factors, including infections, certain drugs (both over-the-counter and prescription), consumption of specific foods and beverages, changes in weather or temperature, aging, hormonal changes or pregnancy, consumption of alcoholic beverages (particularly red wine), nasal inflammation or irritation unrelated to allergies, and symptoms related to other medical disorders. Understanding these factors can aid in the diagnosis and management of non-allergic rhinitis.

Are there any related factors or circumstances?

- Various conditions, depending on the type of rhinitis, may be associated, such as:

- - Asthma, a chronic respiratory condition characterized by inflammation and narrowing of the airways, often co-occurs with allergic rhinitis due to shared underlying mechanisms of inflammation and immune dysregulation.

- - Acute sinusitis, an inflammation of the nasal sinuses often caused by viral or bacterial infections, can exacerbate symptoms of allergic rhinitis and vice versa, leading to increased nasal congestion and discomfort.

- - Ocular inflammation, known as conjunctivitis or pink eye, frequently accompanies allergic rhinitis, with symptoms including redness, itching, and excessive tearing due to shared allergic triggers affecting both the nasal and ocular mucosa.

- - Eczema or atopic dermatitis, a chronic inflammatory skin condition, commonly coexists with allergic rhinitis, suggesting a potential common underlying immune dysfunction or genetic predisposition.

- - Inadequate ear ventilation, also known as eustachian tube dysfunction, can occur alongside allergic rhinitis, contributing to symptoms such as ear pressure, pain, and impaired hearing due to impaired equalization of middle ear pressure.

- • - Laryngitis, characterized by inflammation of the larynx or voice box, may occur concurrently with allergic rhinitis, leading to symptoms such as hoarseness, throat discomfort, and difficulty speaking.

- • - Eosinophilic esophagitis, a chronic immune-mediated condition characterized by inflammation of the esophagus, shares underlying allergic mechanisms with allergic rhinitis, suggesting potential comorbidity and interconnected pathophysiology.

- • - Sleep deprivation, resulting from nighttime symptoms such as nasal congestion, snoring, and difficulty breathing, often accompanies allergic rhinitis, leading to impaired sleep quality, daytime fatigue, and cognitive dysfunction.

- These associated conditions underscore the systemic nature of allergic rhinitis and its potential impact on various organ systems beyond the nasal cavity. Understanding these interconnections is crucial for comprehensive management and treatment approaches aimed at addressing both the nasal and extranasal manifestations of allergic rhinitis for improved patient outcomes and quality of life.

CHAPTER 3
WHY IS IT ESSENTIAL TO ADDRESS HAY FEVER?

Rhinitis, often perceived as a minor inconvenience, has garnered attention from researchers due to its significant impact on quality of life. Studies have elucidated its disruptive effects on various aspects of daily functioning, including sleep patterns, attention span, and the ability to engage in activities throughout the day. Individuals afflicted with rhinitis frequently find themselves compelled to miss work or school, and the condition has been correlated with diminished academic performance as reflected in test scores.

Furthermore, there exists a noteworthy association between allergic rhinitis and the development of asthma, as the upper airway influences the lower airway leading to the lungs. It's not uncommon for individuals with asthma to also experience rhinitis, often stemming from an allergic reaction. However, it's worth noting that adequately treating rhinitis can contribute to better asthma management, potentially resulting in fewer visits to Accident & Emergency departments or hospitals.

The interconnected nature of rhinitis and asthma underscores the importance of addressing both conditions comprehensively to optimize health outcomes. By managing rhinitis effectively, individuals can potentially mitigate the severity of asthma symptoms and reduce the frequency of exacerbations, thereby enhancing overall respiratory health and quality of life.

Furthermore, beyond the physiological manifestations, allergic rhinitis and its associated symptoms can exert a significant toll on mental well-being, contributing to feelings of frustration, fatigue, and impaired cognitive function. Consequently, comprehensive management approaches should encompass not only pharmacological interventions but also strategies aimed at improving coping mechanisms and enhancing overall resilience.

In light of the multifaceted impact of rhinitis, efforts to raise awareness about the condition and its implications are essential. Educating healthcare professionals, patients, and the general public about the interconnectedness of rhinitis with other respiratory conditions like asthma can foster early detection, prompt intervention, and improved outcomes for affected individuals.

In summary, while rhinitis may sometimes be perceived as a minor ailment, its far-reaching effects on various facets of life underscore the importance of recognizing and addressing it comprehensively. By adopting a holistic approach to management that considers both physiological and psychological aspects, individuals can strive towards better symptom control, enhanced quality of life, and improved overall well-being.

Identifying Allergic Rhinitis

During a medical consultation, a physician might inquire extensively about the onset and severity of allergic rhinitis symptoms, aiming to gain a comprehensive understanding of the patient's condition. Additionally, they may seek to ascertain whether the allergic rhinitis is perennial, persisting throughout the year, or seasonal, occurring mainly during specific times of the year. This detailed inquiry enables the doctor to tailor treatment strategies accordingly to address the patient's unique needs.

In the process of diagnosis, the physician may conduct a thorough examination of the nasal passages to assess any signs of inflammation or irritation. Furthermore, they might consider conducting blood tests to detect the presence of antibodies, providing valuable insights into the immune response and identifying potential allergens triggering the allergic rhinitis.

In cases where allergic rhinitis significantly impairs the patient's quality of life and daily functioning, the physician may refer them to an allergy specialist for further evaluation and management. These specialists possess expertise in diagnosing and treating allergic conditions, employing specialized diagnostic techniques to identify specific allergens responsible for triggering the symptoms.

One of the primary diagnostic tools employed by allergy specialists is the skin prick test, a procedure designed to determine an individual's sensitivity to various allergens. During this test, small amounts of suspected allergens are applied to the skin's surface through gentle pricks or scratches. The skin's reaction to these allergens is then observed, with the appearance of redness, swelling, or itching indicating a positive allergic response.

Additionally, allergy experts may utilize other diagnostic modalities, such as blood tests or nasal endoscopy, to further evaluate the patient's condition and identify potential triggers for allergic rhinitis. These comprehensive diagnostic approaches enable healthcare providers to develop personalized treatment plans tailored to the patient's specific allergies and medical history.

Overall, seeking medical attention from qualified healthcare professionals is essential for accurate diagnosis and effective management of allergic rhinitis. Through thorough evaluation and specialized testing, physicians and allergy specialists can provide targeted interventions to alleviate symptoms and improve the patient's quality of life.

CHAPTER 4
RISK FACTORS FOR ALLERGIC RHINITIS

The risk of developing allergic rhinitis tends to be more pronounced in individuals who have a familial background marked by allergic rhinitis, eczema, or asthma. This familial predisposition suggests a genetic component to the condition, wherein the presence of allergic diseases within the family lineage can increase the likelihood of developing allergic rhinitis. The shared genetic factors among family members can contribute to the inheritance of allergic tendencies, thereby heightening the susceptibility to nasal allergies.

- Furthermore, individuals with a personal history of asthma or eczema are also at an increased risk of experiencing allergic rhinitis. Asthma, a chronic respiratory condition characterized by airway inflammation and constriction, shares common underlying mechanisms with allergic rhinitis, such as immune system dysregulation and heightened sensitivity to allergens. Similarly, eczema, a chronic skin condition characterized by inflammation and itching, is often associated with allergic reactions and may coexist with allergic rhinitis due to shared allergic triggers.

- In addition to familial and personal medical histories, allergies to certain foods can also contribute to an increased risk of allergic rhinitis. The immune system's response to ingested allergens may manifest as allergic rhinitis symptoms, particularly in individuals with underlying allergic tendencies. Consequently, individuals with food allergies should be vigilant about potential allergic reactions and their association with nasal symptoms.

- Understanding these predisposing factors underscores the importance of proactive management and preventive measures for individuals at risk of allergic rhinitis. By addressing genetic susceptibilities, minimizing exposure to environmental triggers, and adopting appropriate treatment strategies, individuals can effectively manage their allergic rhinitis symptoms and improve their overall quality of life. Moreover, ongoing research into the genetic and environmental determinants of allergic diseases holds promise for the development of personalized interventions and targeted therapies in the future.

Treatment for Allergic Rhinitis

The management of allergic rhinitis encompasses a multifaceted approach, typically categorized into four main strategies aimed at alleviating symptoms and improving quality of life.

1. **Avoidance of Allergens and Irritants:** Allergic rhinitis is often triggered by inhaled allergens such as pollen, dust mites, and animal dander, as well as, in rare cases, by certain food

allergies. While some allergens like pet dander can be avoided, others like pollen pose a greater challenge. Strategies for allergen avoidance may include measures such as using allergen-proof bedding covers, minimizing exposure to soft furnishings and heavy drapes, and opting for hard flooring surfaces. However, the effectiveness of such avoidance techniques in controlled clinical trials remains inconclusive. Additionally, avoiding irritants like cigarette smoke can contribute to symptom relief, while nasal irrigation with a saline solution can provide soothing relief from nasal discomfort.

2. **Medication:** For mild to moderate hay fever symptoms, antihistamines are commonly recommended. It's crucial to opt for non-sedating antihistamines to avoid compromising daily

activities such as driving or work performance. More severe or chronic rhinitis may require treatment with topical nasal corticosteroid sprays or nasal drops, particularly if sinusitis or nasal polyps are present. Nasal corticosteroid sprays, being non-absorbable, are considered safe for both adults and children. However, it may take several days or weeks for symptoms to fully resolve, and combination therapies may be necessary for optimal management. Other potentially effective treatments include anti-leukotriene pills, chromones, and ipratropium.

3. **Immunotherapy:** Immunotherapy, also known as desensitization, involves gradually increasing exposure to allergens to build tolerance and reduce allergic reactions. This long-term approach may offer lasting relief for individuals

who do not respond adequately to other treatment modalities or have specific troublesome allergies. Immunotherapy can be administered via subcutaneous injections or sublingual tablets or drops. While sublingual immunotherapy can be self-administered at home following initial supervision, injectable immunotherapy requires administration by healthcare professionals due to the potential for severe side effects.

4. **Surgical Intervention:** Surgical intervention for allergic rhinitis is rare and typically reserved for cases unresponsive to other treatments or those with structural abnormalities obstructing the nasal passages. Procedures may include surgery with or without turbinate reduction to improve access for topical nasal sprays or to alleviate sinus blockages

in individuals with inadequate response to medical therapy.

In summary, the management of allergic rhinitis involves a comprehensive approach tailored to individual symptoms and needs, encompassing allergen avoidance, medication, immunotherapy, and, in rare cases, surgical intervention. Seeking guidance from healthcare professionals is essential to ensure appropriate treatment selection and management of symptoms for optimal relief and improved quality of life.

Ginger Glazed Mahi Mahi

Ingredients

- 3 tablespoons honey

- 3 tablespoons soy sauce

- 3 tablespoons balsamic vinegar

- 2 teaspoons olive oil

- 1 teaspoon grated fresh ginger root

- 1 clove garlic, crushed or to taste

- 4 (6 ounce) mahi mahi fillets

- salt and pepper to taste

- 1 tablespoon vegetable oil

How To Make

1. Mix honey, soy sauce, balsamic vinegar, olive oil, ginger, and garlic together in a shallow dish. Season fish fillets with salt and pepper; place them skin-sides down in the dish with marinade. Cover and refrigerate for 20 minutes.

2. Heat vegetable oil in a large skillet over medium-high heat. Remove fish fillets, reserving marinade. Fry fish for 4 to 6 minutes on each side, turning only once, until fish flakes easily with a fork. Remove fillets to a serving platter and keep warm.

3. Pour reserved marinade into the skillet; simmer over medium heat until reduced to a glaze. Spoon glaze over fish and serve.

Sesame-Crusted Mahi Mahi with Soy, Shiso, and Ginger Butter Sauce

Ingredients

- ½ cup dry white wine

- 1 lemon, juiced

- 3 shallots, minced

- 2 teaspoons minced fresh ginger root

- ½ cup heavy cream

- 3 tablespoons soy sauce

- ½ cup unsalted butter, chilled and cut into small cubes

- 4 shiso leaves

- coarse kosher salt

- ground white pepper

- 2 tablespoons canola oil

- 6 (6 ounce) mahi mahi fillets

- 4 tablespoons sesame seeds

- 4 tablespoons black sesame seeds

How To Make

1. Combine white wine, lemon juice, shallots, and ginger in a saucepan over medium heat. Cook until liquid is reduced to approximately 2

tablespoons. Stir in heavy cream and bring to light boil. Reduce cream by half; do not burn. Stir in soy sauce, then transfer to a blender. Blend on low while slowly adding butter, a few cubes at a time, until all of the butter is emulsified. Roughly chop or tear shiso, add to sauce, and blend for about 10 more seconds. Season to taste with salt and white pepper. Keep the sauce warm.

2. Preheat the oven to 425 degrees F (220 degrees C).

3. Heat oil in a large oven-safe sauté pan over high heat. Season both sides of the mahi mahi with salt and white pepper.

4. Mix white and black sesame seeds together on a plate or flat dish. Place the top side only of each fillet into sesame seeds, pressing fillets down into

seeds so they stick. Make sure that the crusted sides are evenly crusted with seeds.

5. Add fish, sesame seed-side down, to the pan once oil is smoking. Be careful of oil splatters. Pan-sear fish for about 30 to 45 seconds per side.

6. Move the pan into the preheated oven, or transfer fish to a baking sheet, and cook for 5 to 6 minutes.

7. Serve fillets, sesame crust-side up, with ginger butter sauce.

Steamed Fish with Ginger

Ingredients

• 1 pound halibut fillet

- 1 teaspoon coarse sea salt or kosher salt

- 1 tablespoon minced fresh ginger

- 3 tablespoons thinly sliced green onion

- 1 tablespoon dark soy sauce

- 1 tablespoon light soy sauce

- 1 tablespoon peanut oil

- 2 teaspoons toasted sesame oil

- ¼ cup lightly packed fresh cilantro sprigs

How To Make

1. Pat halibut dry with paper towels. Rub both sides of fillet with salt. Scatter the ginger over the top of the fish and place onto a heatproof ceramic dish.

2. Place into a bamboo steamer set over several inches of gently boiling water, and cover. Gently steam for 10 to 12 minutes.

3. Pour accumulated water out of the dish and sprinkle the fillet with green onion. Drizzle both soy sauces over the surface of the fish.

4. Heat peanut and sesame oils in a small skillet over medium-high heat until they begin to smoke. When the oil is hot, carefully pour on top of the halibut fillet. The very hot oil will cause the green onions and water on top of the fish to pop and spatter all over; be careful. Garnish with cilantro sprigs and serve immediately.

Garlic-Ginger Chicken Wings

Ingredients

• cooking spray

• 5 pounds chicken wings, separated at joints, tips discarded

• salt and ground black pepper to taste

• 3 tablespoons hot sauce (such as Frank's Red Hot ®)

• 2 tablespoons vegetable oil

• 1 cup all-purpose flour

For the glaze:

• 3 crushed garlic cloves

- 2 tablespoons minced fresh ginger root

- 1 tablespoon Asian chile pepper sauce

- ½ cup rice vinegar

- ½ cup packed brown sugar

- 1 tablespoon soy sauce

How To Make

1. Preheat oven to 400 degrees F (200 degrees C). Line 2 baking sheets with aluminum foil; grease the foil with cooking spray.

2. Place the chicken in a large mixing bowl. Season with salt, pepper, and hot sauce. Add the vegetable oil; toss to coat.

3. Place the flour and wings in a large, food-safe plastic bag. Hold the bag closed tightly, and shake

to coat the wings entirely with the flour; no wet spots should remain. Arrange the wings on the prepared baking sheets, making sure none of the pieces are touching one another. Spray wings with additional cooking spray

4. Bake in the preheated oven for 30 minutes, turn all the wings, and return to the oven to cook until crispy and no longer pink in the center, about 30 minutes more.

5. Whisk together the garlic, ginger, chili paste, rice vinegar, brown sugar, and soy sauce in a saucepan. Bring the mixture to a boil and immediately remove from heat.

6. Put about half the wings in a large mixing bowl. Pour about half the sauce over the wings. Toss the wings with tongs to coat evenly; transfer to a tray and allow to sit about 5 minutes to allow the sauce

to soak into the wings before serving. Repeat with remaining wings and sauce.

Fast Salmon with a Ginger Glaze

Ingredients

- 4 (8 ounce) fresh salmon fillets

- salt to taste

- ⅓ cup cold water

- ¼ cup seasoned rice vinegar

- 2 tablespoons brown sugar

- 1 tablespoon hot chile paste (such as sambal oelek)

- 1 tablespoon finely grated fresh ginger

- 4 cloves garlic, minced

- 1 teaspoon soy sauce

- ¼ cup chopped fresh basil

How To Make

1. Preheat grill for medium heat and lightly oil the grate.

2. Season salmon fillets with salt.

3. Place salmon on the preheated grill; cook salmon for 6 to 8 minutes per side, or until the fish flakes easily with a fork.

4. Combine water, rice vinegar, brown sugar, chile paste, ginger, garlic, and soy sauce in a small saucepan over medium heat.

5. Bring mixture to a boil, reduce heat to medium and simmer until barely thickened, about 2 minutes.

6. Sprinkle basil on top of salmon; spoon glaze over basil.

Thai Ginger Chicken (Gai Pad King)

Ingredients

- 1 ½ cups uncooked jasmine rice

- 3 ½ cups water

- 2 tablespoons vegetable oil

- 3 cloves garlic, minced

- 1 pound skinless, boneless chicken breast halves - cut into thin strips

- 1 tablespoon Asian fish sauce

- 1 tablespoon oyster sauce

- 1 tablespoon white sugar

- ½ cup fresh ginger, cut into matchsticks

- 1 large red bell pepper, cut into strips

- ¾ cup sliced fresh mushrooms

- 4 green onions cut into 2-inch pieces

- ½ teaspoon Thai red chile paste, or to taste

- 2 tablespoons chicken broth

- salt and ground black pepper to taste

• 2 tablespoons fresh cilantro leaves

Ingredients

1. Bring the rice and water to a boil in a saucepan. Reduce heat to medium-low; cover and simmer until the rice is tender and the liquid has been absorbed, 20 to 25 minutes.

2. Meanwhile, heat a wok or large skillet over medium-high heat. Stir in the garlic and chicken; cook for 2 minutes. Add the fish sauce, oyster sauce, sugar, ginger, red pepper, mushrooms, and onions. Cook and stir until the chicken is no longer pink and the vegetables are nearly tender, about 3 minutes. Dissolve the chile paste in the chicken broth, then add to the chicken mixture. Season to taste with salt and pepper; sprinkle with cilantro leaves to garnish. Serve with the hot rice.

Peanut-Ginger Marinade

Ingredients

- ½ cup hot water

- ½ cup creamy peanut butter

- ¼ cup chile paste

- ¼ cup soy sauce

- 2 tablespoons vegetable oil

- 2 tablespoons white vinegar

- 4 cloves garlic, minced

- 2 teaspoons grated fresh ginger root

- ¼ teaspoon ground red pepper

How To Make

1. In a large bowl, gradually stir hot water into peanut butter. Stir in chile paste, soy sauce, oil, vinegar, garlic, ginger, and ground red pepper.

To Use:

Pour marinade into a resealable plastic bag. Add 2 to 3 pounds meat, coat with the marinade, squeeze out excess air, and seal the bag. Marinate in the refrigerator for 8 hours to overnight. Remove meat from the marinade and shake off excess. Discard the remaining marinade. Cook meat as desired.

Best Fried Green Tomatoes

Ingredients

- 4 large green tomatoes

- 2 eggs

- ½ cup milk

- 1 cup all-purpose flour

- ½ cup cornmeal

- ½ cup bread crumbs

- 2 teaspoons coarse kosher salt

- ¼ teaspoon ground black pepper

- 1 quart vegetable oil for frying

How To Make

1. Slice tomatoes 1/2 inch thick. Discard the ends.

2. Whisk eggs and milk together in a medium-size bowl. Scoop flour onto a plate. Mix cornmeal, bread crumbs and salt and pepper on another plate. Dip tomatoes into flour to coat. Then dip the tomatoes into milk and egg mixture. Dredge in breadcrumbs to completely coat.

3. In a large skillet, pour vegetable oil (enough so that there is 1/2 inch of oil in the pan) and heat over a medium heat. Place tomatoes into the frying pan in batches of 4 or 5, depending on the size of your skillet. Do not crowd the tomatoes, they should not touch each other. When the tomatoes are browned, flip and fry them on the other side. Drain them on paper towels.

Spaghetti Sauce with Fresh Tomatoes

Ingredients

- ¼ cup olive oil

- 1 onion, chopped

- ½ teaspoon garlic powder

- 4 pounds fresh tomatoes, peeled and chopped

- 1 tablespoon white sugar

- 1 tablespoon dried basil

- 1 tablespoon dried parsley

- 1 teaspoon salt

How To Make

1. Heat olive oil in a large skillet over medium heat. Add onion and garlic powder; cook and stir until onion is translucent, about 5 minutes.

2. Add tomatoes, sugar, basil, parsley, and salt; bring to a boil. Reduce heat and simmer, stirring occasionally, until sauce thickens, 1 to 2 hours.

Roasted Cherry Tomatoes with Angel Hair

Ingredients

- 1 (10 ounce) basket cherry tomatoes, halved

- 1 tablespoon olive oil

- 1 teaspoon minced garlic

- salt and ground black pepper to taste

- 4 ounces angel hair pasta

- 3 basil leaves, cut into thin strips, or more to taste

- 1 dash red pepper flakes

- 2 tablespoons fresh grated Parmesan cheese, or to taste (Optional)

How To Make

1. Preheat oven to 375 degrees F (190 degrees C).

2. Combine tomatoes, olive oil, garlic, salt, and pepper in a bowl until well mixed; spread on a shallow-sided baking sheet.

3. Bake in the preheated oven until tomatoes are soft and wrinkled, 25 to 30 minutes.

4. Bring a large pot of lightly salted water to a boil. Cook angel hair pasta in the boiling water, stirring

occasionally until tender yet firm to the bite, 4 to 5 minutes. Drain; reserving a small amount of cooking water.

5. Spoon tomatoes with their juices into a small saucepan; add basil and red pepper flakes. Mix in reserved cooking water to thin tomato mixture to desired consistency. Cook and stir over low heat until warmed, about 5 minutes; stir in pasta. Top with Parmesan cheese before serving.

Notes:

Grape tomatoes can be substituted for cherry tomatoes. Chicken stock can be used instead of pasta water to thin tomatoes.

Creamy Pasta Bake with Cherry Tomatoes and Basil

Ingredients

- 1 (16 ounce) package penne pasta

- 1 tablespoon olive oil

- 1 onion, finely chopped

- 3 cloves garlic, minced

- 3 (6 ounce) cans tomato sauce

- 2 tablespoons tomato paste

- ¾ cup heavy whipping cream

- ½ cup grated Parmesan cheese

- 1 pinch white sugar

- salt and freshly ground black pepper

- 1 pound cherry tomatoes, halved

- 1 ¼ cups shredded mozzarella cheese

- 1 small bunch fresh basil, finely chopped

How To Make

1. Preheat the oven to 400 degrees F (200 degrees C). Grease a baking dish.

2. Bring a large pot of lightly salted water to a boil. Add penne and cook, stirring occasionally, until tender yet firm to the bite, about 11 minutes. Drain, reserving 1 cup cooking water.

3. Heat olive oil in a large skillet over medium heat. Cook onion in oil until soft and translucent, about 5 minutes. Add garlic and cook for an additional 30 seconds. Stir in tomato sauce and

tomato paste and cook until slightly reduced, about 5 minutes. Add cream and Parmesan cheese. Season with sugar, salt, and pepper.

4. Stir some of the reserved pasta water into sauce and add cooked penne. Remove from the heat and stir in cherry tomatoes, 1/2 of the mozzarella cheese, and basil. Add more pasta water if needed to reach desired consistency. Pour penne mixture into the prepared baking dish and cover with remaining mozzarella cheese.

5. Bake in the preheated oven until bubbly and cheese is melted, about 20 minutes.

Roasted Tomatoes with Garlic

Ingredients

• 4 cups grape tomatoes

• 4 cloves garlic, sliced

• 2 tablespoons olive oil

• salt and pepper to taste

Ingredients

1. Preheat an oven to 450 degrees F (230 degrees C). Place a piece of aluminum foil over a baking sheet.

2. Place the tomatoes and garlic into a mixing bowl. Drizzle with olive oil, and toss until evenly coated. Season to taste with salt and pepper, then spread evenly onto the prepared baking sheet.

3. Bake the grape tomatoes in the preheated oven until the skins pop and start to brown, 15 to 20 minutes.

Vera Cruz Tomatoes

Ingredients

* 4 firm ripe tomatoes

* 3 slices bacon

* ¼ cup chopped onion

* 8 ounces fresh spinach, stems snipped

* ½ cup sour cream

* ¼ teaspoon hot pepper sauce

* salt to taste

* ½ cup shredded Mexican cheese blend

Ingredients

1. Preheat an oven to 375 degrees F (190 degrees C). Grease an 8x8 inch baking dish.

2. Cut tops from tomatoes; remove seeds and membranes. Place tomato shells upside down on paper towels to drain until filling.

3. Place the bacon in a large, deep skillet, and cook over medium-high heat, turning occasionally, until evenly browned, about 10 minutes. Drain the bacon slices on a paper towel-lined plate, reserve drippings. Crumble bacon and set aside. Return 2 tablespoons of drippings to skillet.

4. Cook onion in the bacon drippings until tender, about 5 minutes. Stir in spinach; cook and stir until wilted, about 2 minutes. Remove from heat. Stir in sour cream, reserved crumbled bacon, and hot pepper sauce.

5. Sprinkle tomato shells with salt; fill evenly with bacon and spinach mixture. Place tomatoes in prepared baking dish.

6. Bake in preheated oven until hot, 20 to 25 minutes. Remove, and top evenly with the shredded cheese. Return to the oven; bake until cheese is melted, about 5 minutes.

Parmesan Tomatoes

Ingredients

• 4 ripe tomatoes, sliced

• 4 tablespoons mayonnaise

• 4 tablespoons Parmesan cheese

- 1 tablespoon Dijon mustard

- 1 tablespoon brown mustard

- 1 teaspoon dried oregano

- salt and pepper to taste

- 1 teaspoon chopped fresh parsley

- ¼ cup shredded mozzarella cheese

Ingredients

1. Preheat oven to 350 degrees F (175 degrees C).

2. Arrange tomato slices in a single layer on a baking sheet. In a small bowl, mix together mayonnaise, parmesan, Dijon mustard, and brown mustard. Season with oregano, and salt and pepper to taste. Use a spoon to top each tomato slice with a small amount of the mayonnaise

mixture. Sprinkle with mozzarella , and then top with parsley.

3. Bake in preheated oven for approximately 15 minutes, or until golden brown. Serve immediately.

Chicken with Artichokes and Sundried Tomatoes

Ingredients

- 2 tablespoons olive oil

- ½ onion, sliced

- 2 cloves garlic, minced

- 1 pound skinless, boneless chicken breast halves, cut into 1-inch pieces

- ½ cup chicken broth

- 1 (15 ounce) can quartered artichoke hearts, undrained

- 1 (6 ounce) jar sun-dried tomatoes, drained and cut into quarters

- 1 (4 ounce) can sliced olives, drained

- 1 teaspoon salt

- ½ teaspoon dried oregano

- ½ teaspoon dried basil

- freshly ground black pepper to taste

- 1 (12 ounce) package angel hair pasta

• 1 (8 ounce) package crumbled feta cheese

How To Make

1. Heat olive oil in a large skillet over medium-high heat; cook and stir onion and garlic in hot oil for 1 minute. Add chicken; cook and stir until chicken is no longer pink, 5 to 10 minutes. Stir chicken broth, artichoke hearts with juice, sun-dried tomatoes, olives, salt, oregano, basil, and black pepper into chicken mixture; cover skillet and simmer until chicken is cooked through, about 10 more minutes.

2. Bring a large pot of lightly salted water to a boil. Cook angel hair in the boiling water, stirring occasionally until cooked through but firm to the bite, 4 to 5 minutes. Drain and transfer pasta to a platter; spoon chicken mixture over pasta. Sprinkle with feta cheese.

Scalloped Tomatoes

Ingredients

- ¼ cup butter

- 1 onion, chopped

- 1 teaspoon salt

- ground black pepper to taste

- ½ teaspoon dried basil

- 4 teaspoons brown sugar

- 5 tomatoes, sliced

- 2 cups white bread cubes

Ingredients

1. Preheat the oven to 375 degrees F (190 degrees C). Grease a 9x13-inch casserole dish.

2. Sauté butter and onion in a medium saucepan over medium heat until onion is translucent, 3 to 4 minutes. Add salt, pepper, basil, brown sugar, and tomatoes; mix well. Stir in bread until well combined. Pour tomato-bread mixture into the prepared dish.

3. Bake in the preheated oven for 30 to 35 minutes. Enjoy.

Okra and Tomatoes

Ingredients

- 2 slices bacon

- 1 pound frozen okra, thawed and sliced

- 1 small onion, chopped

- ½ green bell pepper, chopped

- 2 celery, chopped

- 1 (14.5 ounce) can stewed tomatoes

- salt and pepper to taste

How To Make

1. Place bacon in a large, deep skillet. Cook over medium-high heat until evenly browned and crisp. Drain; crumble bacon onto a plate and set aside.

2. Add okra, onion, pepper, and celery to the pan; sauté until tender. Add tomatoes, salt, and pepper; cook and stir until tomatoes are heated through.

3. Garnish with crumbled bacon.

Soy Ginger Salmon

Ingredients

• 1 pound salmon fillets

• ⅓ cup brown sugar, divided

• 2 teaspoons lemon pepper, divided

• 1 teaspoon garlic powder, divided

• ⅓ cup low sodium soy sauce

- 1 tablespoon olive oil

- 1 (1 inch) piece fresh ginger root, minced

- ⅓ cup orange juice

How To Make

1. Rub salmon with about 1 tablespoon brown sugar. Lightly sprinkle with lemon pepper and garlic powder; rub seasoning into fish.

2. Into a small saucepan set over medium heat, pour soy sauce and olive oil. Stir in ginger and remaining brown sugar, lemon pepper, and garlic powder. Bring to a gentle simmer, stirring constantly until sugar has dissolved. Remove from heat, stir in orange juice.

3. Place fish and marinade into a resealable plastic bag, seal, and refrigerate overnight, or for at least 3 hours.

4. Preheat broiler. Place fish in a foil-lined baking pan. Reserve marinade.

5. Broil fish skin-side up, 2 minutes. Remove from oven, pull skin off with tongs. Baste with marinade, return to oven, and broil 2 minutes more. Turn fish, and broil until fish flakes easily, about 4 minutes. Remove from oven, and let sit 5 minutes before serving.

Chicken Noodle Salad with Peanut-Ginger Dressing

Ingredients

Dressing

- ⅓ cup smooth peanut butter

- ¼ cup soy sauce

- 2 tablespoons unseasoned rice vinegar

- 1 tablespoon Asian garlic-chili sauce

- 1 tablespoon brown sugar, packed

- 1 tablespoon finely chopped fresh ginger root

- ⅛ teaspoon red pepper flakes

- 3 tablespoons low-sodium chicken broth

- salt and ground black pepper to taste

Salad

- 1 (16 ounce) package uncooked linguine pasta

- 3 ½ cups cooked chicken, cut into strips

- 1 cup julienne-sliced carrot

- 6 green onions, chopped

- 1 red bell pepper, seeded and cut into strips

- 1 celery rib, thinly sliced

- ½ cup fresh cilantro leaves, chopped

- ½ cup chopped roasted peanuts, for garnish

Ingredients

1. To make the dressing, place the peanut butter, soy sauce, rice vinegar, chili-garlic sauce, brown sugar, ginger, red pepper flakes, and 3 tablespoons of chicken broth together in a blender or bowl of a food processor. Blend until smooth. Season to taste

with salt and pepper. Thin the dressing to your taste by adding more chicken broth or water.

2. Bring a large pot of lightly salted water to a boil. Add the linguine and cook until al dente, 8 to 10 minutes. Drain and place pasta into a large mixing bowl.

3. Add the chicken, carrots, green onions, red pepper, celery, and cilantro to the bowl with the linguine. Pour the dressing over the noodle-chicken mixture and toss until mixture is evenly coated. Divide the salad among eight serving plates, and sprinkle peanuts over each serving.

Crispy Ginger Beef

Ingredients

- ¾ cup cornstarch

- ½ cup water

- 2 large eggs

- 1 pound flank steak, cut into thin strips

- ½ cup canola oil, or as needed

- 1 large carrot, cut into matchstick-size pieces

- 1 green bell pepper, cut into matchstick-size pieces

- 1 red bell pepper, cut into matchstick-size pieces

- 3 green onions, chopped

- ¼ cup minced fresh ginger root

- 5 garlic cloves, minced

- ½ cup white sugar

- ¼ cup rice vinegar

- 3 tablespoons soy sauce

- 1 tablespoon sesame oil

- 1 tablespoon red pepper flakes, or to taste

Ingredients

1. Place cornstarch in a large bowl; gradually whisk in water until smooth. Whisk eggs into cornstarch mixture; toss steak strips in mixture to coat.

2. Pour canola oil into a wok, 1-inch deep; heat oil over high heat until hot but not smoking. Place 1/4 of the beef strips into hot oil; separate strips with a fork. Cook, stirring frequently, until coating is

crisp and golden, about 3 minutes. Remove beef to drain on paper towels; repeat with remaining beef.

3. Drain off all but 1 tablespoon oil; cook and stir carrot, bell peppers, green onions, ginger, and garlic over high heat until lightly browned but still crisp, about 3 minutes.

4. Whisk sugar, rice vinegar, soy sauce, sesame oil, and red pepper flakes together in a small bowl. Pour sauce mixture over vegetables in wok; bring mixture to a boil. Stir beef back into vegetable mixture; cook and stir just until heated through, about 3 minutes.

Tips

This is the original recipe but I like to add about 1/4 cup of teriyaki sauce as a variation. I also like to add sesame oil to the oil when I fry the beef.

Carrot and Ginger Soup

Ingredients

• ½ medium butternut squash

• 2 tablespoons olive oil

• 1 onion, diced

• 1 pound carrots - peeled and diced

• 3 cloves garlic, crushed or to taste

• 1 (2 inch) piece fresh ginger, peeled and thinly sliced

• 4 cups water

• salt and pepper to taste

• 1 pinch ground cinnamon

• ¼ cup heavy cream (Optional)

Ingredients

1. Preheat the oven to 350 degrees F (175 degrees C). Scoop seeds out of the butternut squash half, and place cut side down onto a greased baking sheet. Bake for 30 to 40 minutes, or until softened. Allow to cool, then scoop the squash flesh out of the skin using a large spoon and set aside. Discard skin.

2. Heat olive oil in a large saucepan or soup pot over medium heat. Add chopped onion and garlic, and cook, stirring until onion is translucent. Pour in the water, and add squash, carrots and ginger. Bring to a boil, and cook for at least 20 minutes, or until carrots and ginger are tender.

3. Puree the mixture in the blender, or using an immersion blender. Add boiling water if necessary to thin, but bear in mind this is meant to be a thick creamy soup. Return soup to the pan, and heat through. Season with salt, pepper and cinnamon.

4. Ladle into serving bowls, and pour a thin swirl of cream over the top as a garnish if desired.

Ginger Veggie Stir-Fry

Ingredients

• 4 tablespoons vegetable oil, divided

• 2 teaspoons chopped fresh ginger root, divided

• 1 ½ cloves garlic, crushed

- 1 tablespoon cornstarch

- 1 small head broccoli, cut into florets

- ¾ cup julienned carrots

- ½ cup snow peas

- ½ cup halved green beans

- 2 ½ tablespoons water

- 2 tablespoons soy sauce

- ¼ cup chopped onion

- ½ tablespoon salt

Ingredients

1. Place 2 tablespoons vegetable oil, 1 teaspoon ginger, garlic, and cornstarch in a large bowl; mix

until cornstarch is dissolved. Add broccoli, carrots, snow peas, and green beans; toss lightly to coat.

2. Heat remaining 2 tablespoons vegetable oil in a large skillet or wok over medium heat. Add vegetable mixture and cook for 2 minutes, stirring constantly to prevent burning.

3. Stir in water and soy sauce; add onion, salt, and remaining 1 teaspoon ginger. Cook and stir until vegetables are tender but crisp.

Rib-Eye Steaks with a Soy and Ginger Marinade

Ingredients

- ½ cup soy sauce

- ¼ cup real maple syrup

- 6 cloves garlic, minced

- 1 tablespoon grated fresh ginger

- 1 teaspoon mustard powder

- ½ teaspoon sesame oil

- ¼ teaspoon hot pepper sauce

- ½ cup beer

- 4 (10 ounce) beef rib-eye steaks

How To Make

1. Combine soy sauce, maple syrup, garlic, ginger, mustard powder, sesame oil, and hot pepper sauce in a medium mixing bowl; mix well to blend. Add beer and stir lightly to mix.

2. Prepare steaks by scoring any fatty outside areas on steak with a knife (this prevents the steaks from curling when grilling). Place steaks in a casserole dish and pour marinade over. Using a fork, punch holes in steaks so that the marinade penetrates into the meat. Turn steaks over and repeat punching holes.

3. Cover with clear wrap or foil and let marinate in the refrigerator for 1 hour to overnight.

4. Prepare and preheat a grill to high heat. Place steaks directly on the grill and sear one side for about 15 seconds. Turn steaks over and cook for about 5 minutes, then turn over and cook for another 5 minutes for medium-rare, depending on thickness. Test for doneness by cutting into the middle of the steak.

Adobo Chicken with Ginger

Ingredients

• 1 (3 pound) whole chicken, cut into 8 pieces

• ¾ cup distilled white vinegar

• ½ cup soy sauce

• 2 tablespoons thinly sliced fresh ginger root

• ½ tablespoon black peppercorns

• 1 bulb garlic, peeled and crushed

• 2 bay leaves

Ingredients

1. Combine chicken, vinegar, soy sauce, ginger, peppercorns, garlic, and bay leaves in a Dutch

oven; bring to a boil over medium heat. Reduce heat, cover, and simmer for 30 minutes, basting chicken occasionally with the sauce.

2. Remove the lid and continue to simmer until liquid has reduced by half, 5 to 10 minutes. An instant-read thermometer inserted near the bone should read 165 degrees F (74 degrees C).

3. Transfer chicken to a serving plate. Strain liquid from the pot to remove bay leaves and other solids.

4. Serve chicken hot and drizzle with strained sauce.

Baked Sweet Potatoes with Ginger and Honey

Ingredients

- 3 pounds sweet potatoes, peeled and cubed

- ½ cup honey

- 3 tablespoons grated fresh ginger

- 2 tablespoons walnut oil

- 1 teaspoon ground cardamom

- ½ teaspoon ground black pepper

How To Make

1. Preheat the oven to 400 degrees F (200 degrees C).

2. Toss sweet potatoes, honey, ginger, oil, cardamom, and pepper together in a large bowl. Transfer to a large cast iron skillet.

3. Bake in the preheated oven until sweet potatoes are tender and caramelized, about 40 minutes, stirring halfway through.

Honey Ginger Carrots

Ingredients

• 1 pound carrots, sliced

• ¼ cup butter

• 2 ½ tablespoons honey

• 1 pinch ground ginger

• 1 tablespoon lemon juice, or to taste

Ingredients

1. Bring a pot of water to a boil. Add carrots and cook until tender but still firm, about 5 minutes. Drain.

2. In a large skillet over low heat, melt butter with honey. Stir in ground ginger and lemon juice. Stir in carrots and simmer until heated through.

Stir-Fry Pork with Ginger

Ingredients

• 2 tablespoons vegetable oil

• ½ inch piece fresh ginger root, thinly sliced

• ¼ pound thinly sliced lean pork

• 1 teaspoon soy sauce

- ½ teaspoon dark soy sauce

- ½ teaspoon salt

- ⅓ teaspoon sugar

- 1 teaspoon sesame oil

- 1 green onion, chopped

- 1 tablespoon Chinese rice wine

Ingredients

1. Heat oil in a large skillet or wok over medium-high heat. Fry ginger in hot oil until fragrant, then add pork, soy sauce, dark soy sauce, salt, and sugar. Cook, stirring occasionally, for 10 minutes.

2. Stir in the sesame oil, green onion, and rice wine. Simmer until the pork is tender.

Ginger Pork

Ingredients

- 1 pound boneless pork loin, cubed

- ½ cup all-purpose flour

- 1 ½ tablespoons peanut oil

- ¼ cup chicken broth

- ¼ cup water, or more as needed

- 2 tablespoons soy sauce

- 1 tablespoon sherry

- 2 tablespoons thinly sliced green onion

- 1 clove garlic, minced

- 1 teaspoon white sugar

- 1 teaspoon ground ginger

- salt and pepper to taste

Ingredients

1. Combine cubed pork and flour in a resealable plastic bag. Seal the bag and shake until pork is coated.

2. Heat oil in a large skillet or wok. Add coated pork and brown quickly, about 5 minutes. Transfer pork with a slotted spoon to a bowl; discard remaining oil from the skillet.

3. Add chicken broth, 1/4 cup water, soy sauce, and sherry to the skillet. Stir in green onion, garlic, sugar, ginger, salt, and pepper. Add pork cubes

and bring to a boil. Reduce the heat, cover, and simmer until pork is tender, about 15 minutes. Check occasionally to make sure sauce is not thickening too much. If needed, add more water.

Ginger Salmon

Ingredients

- 2 teaspoons olive oil

- 1 tablespoon honey

- 1 tablespoon Dijon mustard

- 2 teaspoons grated fresh ginger

- 1 pound salmon fillets

How To Make

1. Preheat oven to 350 degrees F (175 degrees C).

2. In a small bowl, blend olive oil, honey, Dijon mustard and ginger

3. Brush salmon fillets evenly with the olive oil mixture. Place in a medium baking dish. Bake 15 to 20 minutes in the preheated oven, until the fish flakes easily with a fork.

Pumpkin Roll with Ginger and Pecans

Ingredients

- 3 eggs

- 1 cup white sugar

- ⅔ cup solid pack pumpkin puree

- 1 teaspoon lemon juice

- ¾ cup all-purpose flour

- 1 teaspoon baking powder

- ½ teaspoon salt

- 2 teaspoons ground cinnamon

- 1 teaspoon ground ginger

- 1 cup chopped pecans

- confectioners' sugar for dusting

- 1 (8 ounce) package cream cheese

- 4 tablespoons butter

- 1 cup confectioners' sugar

- ½ teaspoon vanilla extract

• confectioners' sugar for dusting

Ingredients

1. Preheat oven to 350 degrees F (175 degrees C). Grease and flour a 10x15 inch jellyroll pan.

2. In a large bowl, beat eggs and sugar with an electric mixer on high speed for five minutes. Gradually mix in pumpkin and lemon juice. Combine the flour, baking powder, salt, cinnamon, and ginger; stir into the pumpkin mixture. Spread batter evenly into the prepared pan. Sprinkle pecans over the top of the batter.

3. Bake for 12 to 15 minutes, or until the center springs back when touched. Loosen edges with a knife. Turn out on two dishtowels that have been dusted with confectioners' sugar. Roll up cake using towels, and let cool for about 20 minutes.

4. In a medium bowl, combine cream cheese, butter, 1 cup confectioners' sugar, and vanilla. Beat until smooth. Unroll pumpkin cake when cool, spread with filling, and roll up. Place pumpkin roll on a long sheet of waxed paper, and dust with confectioners' sugar. Wrap cake in waxed paper, and twist ends of waxed paper like a candy wrapper. Refrigerate overnight. Serve chilled; before slicing, dust with additional confectioners' sugar.

Honey-Ginger Grilled Salmon

Ingredients

- 1 teaspoon ground ginger

- 1 teaspoon garlic powder

- ⅓ cup soy sauce

- ⅓ cup orange juice

- ¼ cup honey

- 1 green onion, chopped

- 1 (1 1/2-pound) salmon fillet

How To Make

1. In a large self-closing plastic bag, combine ginger, garlic, soy sauce, orange juice, honey, and green onion; mix well. Place salmon in bag and seal tightly. Turn bag gently to distribute marinade. Refrigerate for 15 to 30 minutes.

2. Preheat an outdoor grill for medium heat and lightly oil grate.

3. Remove salmon from marinade, shake off excess, and discard remaining marinade. Grill for 12 to 15 minutes per inch of thickness, or until the fish flakes easily with a fork.

Grilled Asian Ginger Pork Chops

Ingredients

- ½ cup orange juice

- 2 tablespoons soy sauce

- 2 tablespoons minced fresh ginger root

- 2 tablespoons grated orange zest

- 1 teaspoon minced garlic

- 1 teaspoon garlic chile paste

- ½ teaspoon salt

- 6 pork loin chops, 1/2 inch thick

Ingredients

1. In a shallow container, mix together orange juice, soy sauce, ginger, orange zest, garlic, chile paste, and salt. Add pork chops, and turn to coat evenly. Cover, and refrigerate for at least 2 hours, or overnight. Turn the pork chops in the marinade occasionally.

2. Preheat grill for high heat, and lightly oil grate.

3. Grill pork chops for 5 to 6 minutes per side, or to desired doneness.

Utokia's Ginger Shrimp and Broccoli with Garlic

Ingredients

• Reynolds Parchment Paper

• 4 cups broccoli florets

• 1 pound raw shrimp, peeled and deveined

• 2 cloves garlic, crushed

• 1 tablespoon sesame oil

• ½ tablespoon grated fresh ginger

• ½ tablespoon soy sauce

How To Make

1. Preheat oven to 400 degrees F. Tear off four 15-inch sheets of Reynolds Parchment Paper. Fold

each sheet in half and crease it in the center. Cut each into a heart shape; unfold.

2. Divide broccoli and shrimp evenly on one-half of each sheet near crease.

3. Mix garlic, sesame oil, ginger and soy sauce. Spoon 1/4 the mixture evenly over broccoli and shrimp on each sheet.

4. Fold over other half of each sheet to enclose ingredients. Starting at top, make small overlapping folds down entire length of parchment to secure edges together. Twist last fold several times to make a tight seal. Place parchment packets on a large baking sheet with 1-inch sides.

5. Bake 13 to 15 minutes or until shrimp is done.

6. Place parchment packets on dinner plates. Carefully cut an X in the top of each packet; open

carefully, allowing steam to escape. Serve immediately.

Citrus Swordfish with Citrus Salsa

Ingredients

Salsa:

• 1 medium orange, peeled, sectioned, and cut into bite-size

• ½ cup canned pineapple chunks, undrained

• ¼ cup diced fresh mango

• 2 medium jalapeno peppers, seeded and minced

• 3 tablespoons orange juice

- 1 tablespoon diced red bell pepper

- 2 teaspoons white sugar

- 1 tablespoon chopped fresh cilantro

Swordfish:

- ½ cup fresh orange juice

- 1 tablespoon olive oil

- 1 tablespoon pineapple juice concentrate, thawed

- ¼ teaspoon cayenne pepper

- 1 ½ pounds swordfish steaks

How To Make

1. Make the salsa: Mix orange, pineapple, mango, jalapeños, orange juice, bell pepper, sugar, and

cilantro together in a medium bowl until well combined. Cover and refrigerate until needed.

2. Marinate the swordfish: Whisk orange juice, oil, pineapple juice concentrate, and cayenne together in a large glass or ceramic bowl. Add swordfish and turn to evenly coat. Cover the bowl with plastic wrap and marinate in the refrigerator for 30 minutes.

3. Preheat an outdoor grill for medium-high heat and lightly oil the grate.

4. Remove swordfish from marinade and shake off excess. Discard remaining marinade.

5. Grill on the preheated grill until opaque in the center, 6 to 8 minutes per side. Serve with the salsa.

Citrus Turkey Brine

Ingredients

• 1 (12 pound) fresh, whole, bone-in skin-on turkey, rinsed and patted dry

• 1 cup salt

• 1 medium onion, cut into wedges

• 1 medium orange, cut into wedges

• 1 medium lemon, cut into wedges

• 3 cloves garlic

• 4 large bay leaves

• 1 tablespoon dried thyme

• 1 tablespoon ground black pepper

• 1 ½ gallons cold water

Ingredients

1. Rub turkey all over with salt. Place remaining salt into a large stainless steel or enameled stockpot.

2. Add onion, orange, and lemon wedges to the pot, along with garlic, bay leaves, thyme, and pepper. Place turkey into the pot and pour in cold water. Cover and refrigerate, 8 hours to overnight.

3. When ready to cook, discard brine. Rinse turkey, then pat dry and place in a roasting pan. Refrigerate, uncovered, for 2 to 3 hours. Roast, grill, or deep-fry turkey according to your favorite recipe.

Notes:

Always brine foods in a food-grade, nonreactive container such as a stainless steel or enameled stockpot, a brining bag, or a food-grade plastic bucket.

Easy Garlic Ginger Chicken

Ingredients

- 4 skinless, boneless chicken breast halves

- 3 cloves crushed garlic

- 3 tablespoons ground ginger

- 1 tablespoon olive oil

- 4 limes, juiced

How To Make

1. Pound the chicken to 1/2 inch thickness. In a large resealable plastic bag combine the garlic, ginger, oil and lime juice. Seal bag and shake until blended. Open bag and add chicken. Seal bag and marinate in refrigerator for no more than 20 minutes.

2. Remove chicken from bag and grill or broil, basting with marinade, until cooked through and juices run clear. Dispose of any remaining marinade.

Pork, Apple, and Ginger Stir-Fry with Hoisin Sauce

Ingredients

• 2 tablespoons hoisin sauce

- 2 tablespoons brown sugar

- 6 tablespoons soy sauce

- ½ cup applesauce

- 1 pound pork loin, sliced and cut into thin strips

- 1 ½ tablespoons cornstarch

- 2 tablespoons peanut oil

- ½ teaspoon sesame oil

- 1 tablespoon chopped fresh ginger root

- 3 cups broccoli florets

How To Make

1. Whisk together the hoisin sauce, brown sugar, soy sauce, and applesauce in a small bowl; set aside.

2. Combine the pork and cornstarch in a bowl. Mix until the cornstarch evenly coats the pork; set aside.

3. Heat the peanut oil and sesame oil in a large skillet or wok over medium-high heat. Cook the pork in three separate batches in the hot oil until no longer pink in the middle, 2 to 3 minutes per batch. Remove pork to a plate lined with paper towels to drain, reserving the oil. Add the ginger to the skillet; cook and stir for 30 seconds. Stir in the broccoli and cook until tender. Return the pork to the skillet and pour in the sauce; toss to coat. Cook until all ingredients are hot.

Grilled Ginger-Peanut Pork Tenderloin

Ingredients

- 2 (16 ounce) pork tenderloins, trimmed of fat

- 3 tablespoons soy sauce

- 1 ½ teaspoons sugar or sugar substitute

- 1 tablespoon sesame oil

- 1 tablespoon smooth natural peanut butter

- 1 clove garlic, minced

- 1 teaspoon curry powder

- 1 tablespoon minced fresh ginger

- ½ teaspoon salt

How To Make

1. Place pork in a large resealable plastic bag. Mix together soy sauce, sugar, sesame oil, peanut butter, garlic, curry powder, ginger, and salt in a

bowl until smooth. Pour marinade over tenderloins, press air out of bag, seal, and refrigerate overnight.

2. Preheat an outdoor grill for high heat.

3. Use a paper towel to pat any excess marinade from the pork; allow to sit at room temperature while the grill is heating. Lightly oil grill grate. Cook pork 3 minutes on each side (on all four sides) for a total of 12 to 15 minutes. The pork will be done when it is no longer pink inside and has reached an internal temperature of 145 degrees F (65 degrees C). Remove from the grill and cover meat loosely with a foil tent. Let rest 5 minutes before serving.

Ginger Rhubarb Crisp

Ingredients

- 1 cup white sugar

- 3 tablespoons all-purpose flour

- ½ teaspoon salt

- 2 beaten eggs

- zest from 1 orange

- 2 tablespoons grated fresh ginger root

- 8 cups chopped rhubarb

- ½ cup all-purpose flour

- 2 cups brown sugar

- ½ cup salted butter

- 2 teaspoons cinnamon

- 2 cups rolled oats

How To Make

1. Move an oven rack to the center of oven and preheat oven to 350 degrees F (175 degrees C). Grease a 9x13-inch baking dish.

2. Mix the white sugar, 3 tablespoons of flour, salt, eggs, orange zest, and ginger together in a bowl until well combined; stir in the rhubarb. Pour the rhubarb mixture into the bottom of the prepared baking dish.

3. Thoroughly combine 1/2 cup flour, brown sugar, butter, and cinnamon by pulsing in a food processor or blender. Stir in the oatmeal; crumble

the oatmeal mixture over the rhubarb. Gently pat the topping down to make a crust.

4. Bake on the center rack of preheated oven until the topping is lightly golden, the rhubarb has fallen apart, and the juices are very thick and bubbling, 40 to 50 minutes. Check frequently after 30 minutes to see if bubbles are thick.

Chicken Strawberry Spinach Salad with Ginger-Lime Dressing

Ingredients

• 2 teaspoons corn oil

• 1 skinless, boneless chicken breast half - cut into bite-size pieces

- ½ teaspoon garlic powder

- 1 ½ tablespoons mayonnaise

- ½ lime, juiced

- ½ teaspoon ground ginger

- 2 teaspoons milk

- 2 cups fresh spinach, stems removed

- 4 fresh strawberries, sliced

- 1 ½ tablespoons slivered almonds

- freshly ground black pepper to taste

Ingredients

1. Heat oil in a skillet over medium heat. Place chicken in skillet, season with garlic powder and

cook 10 minutes on each side or until juices run clear. Set aside.

2. In a bowl, mix mayonnaise, lime juice, ginger and milk.

3. Arrange spinach on serving dishes. Top with chicken and strawberries, sprinkle with almonds and drizzle with dressing. Season with pepper to serve.

Cold-Busting Ginger Chicken Noodle Soup

Ingredients

- 1 ½ tablespoons olive oil

- 3 large chicken breasts

* 1 large onion, diced

* 3 cloves garlic, crushed

* 13 cups water

* 2 cups white wine

* ¾ cup fresh lemon juice

* 1 (4 inch) piece fresh ginger, peeled and thinly sliced

* 7 whole black peppercorns

* 4 cubes chicken bouillon

* 3 bay leaves

* 1 tablespoon white sugar

* ¾ cup peeled and sliced carrots

- 2 stalks celery, diced

- 1 kohlrabi bulb, peeled and diced

- 2 ½ tablespoons fresh rosemary

- 2 tablespoons fresh thyme

- 1 (8 ounce) package egg noodles

- 1 large clove garlic, minced

- 1 tablespoon grated ginger

- 1 teaspoon salt, or to taste

- ½ cup chopped fresh parsley

Ingredients

1. Heat olive oil in a large pot over medium heat. Add chicken, onion, and crushed garlic cloves; cook in hot oil until chicken breast is browned and

onions start to turn translucent, about 5 minutes . Pour water, white wine, and lemon juice over the chicken mixture; stir sliced ginger, peppercorns, chicken bouillon, bay leaves, and white sugar into the liquid. Bring to a simmer, reduce heat to medium-low, and cook for 45 minutes.

2. Remove and discard the crushed garlic cloves. Remove chicken breasts from the soup to a cutting board; chop into bite-size pieces.

3. Add carrot, celery, kohlrabi, rosemary, and thyme to the soup. Reduce heat to low until the vegetables begin to soften, about 20 minutes.

4. Bring the soup to a boil. Return chopped chicken to the soup along with the egg noodles, minced garlic, and grated ginger; remove the pot from heat and let sit until the noodles have softened, about 10 minutes. Season with salt. Garnish with parsley.

Roasted Salmon with Orange-Ginger Glaze

Ingredients

• 2 pounds salmon fillet

• 1 cup orange juice

• 2 teaspoons balsamic vinegar

• 1 teaspoon finely chopped fresh ginger root

• salt and ground black pepper to taste

Ingredients

1. Preheat oven to 400 degrees F (200 degrees C).

2. Place orange juice in a small saucepan over medium low heat. Cook and stir 10 to 15 minutes,

until reduced by about 1/2 and thickened. Remove from heat, and allow to cool.

3. Stir balsamic vinegar and ginger root into orange juice.

4. Line a medium baking dish with parchment paper. Place salmon fillet on paper, skin side down. Season with salt and pepper. Cover with 1/2 the orange juice mixture.

5. Bake salmon in the preheated oven 10 to 15 minutes. Brush with remaining marinade, and continue baking 10 to 15 minutes, until easily flaked with a fork

Duck with Honey, Soy, and Ginger

Ingredients

- 2 duck breast halves

- 1 pinch salt

- 1 pinch cayenne pepper

- 1 pinch ground black pepper

- ½ cup chicken stock

- 2 tablespoons honey

- 2 tablespoons soy sauce

- 2 tablespoons rice wine

- 1 tablespoon grated fresh ginger

- 1 tablespoon tomato sauce

- 1 pinch chili powder

- 1 teaspoon lime juice

Ingredients

1. Preheat oven to 400 degrees F (200 degrees C).

2. Use a sharp knife to score across the duck breasts 4 times through the skin and fat but just barely to the meat. Rub the skin with salt, cayenne, and black pepper.

3. Preheat an ovenproof skillet over medium-high heat. Lay the breasts in the skillet skin-side down and fry until the skin is brown and crisp, about 5 minutes. Use a spoon to carefully discard any excess fat from the bottom of the skillet. Turn the breasts over and cook for 1 minute.

4. Place the skillet into the preheated oven and roast until the internal temperature of the thickest part of the breasts reach 160 degrees F (71 degrees C) for well done, or the breasts reach desired doneness.

5. Remove the duck breasts from the skillet and cover with foil. Set aside to rest. Pour off excess fat from the skillet. Place the stock, honey, soy sauce, rice wine, ginger, tomato sauce, chili powder, and lime juice in the skillet. Whisk the sauce over high heat, bring to a boil and cook until the sauce thickens, about 2 minutes. Slice the duck breasts thinly, arrange on serving plates, and pour the sauce over the top.

Marinated Pork Medallions with a Ginger-Apple Compote

Ingredients

- 2 cups balsamic vinegar

- 2 tablespoons minced garlic

- 1 tablespoon chopped fresh thyme

- 1 cup olive oil

- 1 pork tenderloin, cut into 2 inch pieces

- ½ cup butter

- ¼ cup packed brown sugar

- 1 apple, thinly sliced

- ¼ cup dried cherries

- 1 tablespoon minced fresh ginger root

- 1 pinch ground cinnamon

- 1 pinch ground nutmeg

Ingredients

1. Puree the balsamic vinegar, garlic, and thyme in a blender until mixed. With the blender running, slowly pour in the olive oil until thickened and incorporated. Pour the marinade into a resealable plastic bag. Add the pork pieces, coat with the marinade, squeeze out excess air, and seal the bag. Marinate in the refrigerator for 30 minutes.

2. Preheat an outdoor grill for medium heat, and lightly oil the grate. Remove the pork from the marinade, and shake off excess. Discard the remaining marinade.

3. Cook the pork on the preheated grill until no longer pink in the center, about 10 minutes. An instant-read thermometer inserted into the center should read 145 degrees F (63 degrees C). Once cooked, remove from the grill, cover with aluminum foil, and allow to rest for 5 to 10 minutes before slicing.

4. While the pork is cooking, melt the butter in a saucepan over medium heat. Stir in the brown sugar until it begins to simmer. Add the apples, cherries, ginger, cinnamon, and nutmeg. Cook and stir until the apple is tender, about 5 minutes.

Garlic Ginger Tofu

Ingredients

• 3 tablespoons canola oil

• 2 teaspoons minced garlic

• 2 teaspoons minced fresh ginger root

• 1 lime

• 1 tablespoon tamari, or to taste

- 2 pounds firm tofu

Ingredients

1. Heat oil in a wok or skillet over medium heat. Stir in garlic and ginger, and cook for 1 minute. Add tofu to the pan with tamari, and stir to coat. Cover, and continue cooking for 20 to 30 minutes.

2. Squeeze lime juice over tofu before serving.

Candied Citrus Peel

Ingredients

- 1 cup orange peel, cut into strips

- ½ cup white sugar

- ¼ cup water

Ingredients

1. Place peel strips in large saucepan and cover with water. Bring to a boil over high heat, then reduce heat and simmer 10 minutes longer. Drain. Repeat this process two more times.

2. In a medium saucepan, heat sugar and 1/4 cup water over high heat until boiling. Place peel in sugar mixture, reduce heat and simmer 15 minutes, until sugar is dissolved. Remove peel with slotted spoon and dry on wire rack overnight. Store in airtight container.

Orange, Walnut, Gorgonzola and Mixed Greens Salad with Fresh Citrus Vinaigrette

Ingredients

- ¾ cup walnut halves

- 10 ounces mixed salad greens with arugula

- 2 large navel oranges, peeled and sectioned

- ½ cup sliced red onion

- ¼ cup olive oil

- ¼ cup vegetable oil

- ⅔ cup orange juice

- ¼ cup white sugar

- 2 tablespoons balsamic vinegar

- 2 teaspoons Dijon mustard

- ¼ teaspoon dried oregano

- ¼ teaspoon ground black pepper

* ¼ cup crumbled Gorgonzola cheese

Ingredients

1. Place the walnuts in a skillet over medium heat. Cook 5 minutes, stirring constantly, until lightly browned.

2. In a large bowl, toss the toasted walnuts, salad greens, oranges, and red onion.

3. In a large jar with a lid, mix the olive oil, vegetable oil, orange juice, sugar, vinegar, mustard, oregano, and pepper. Seal jar, and shake to mix.

4. Divide the salad greens mixture into individual servings. To serve, sprinkle with Gorgonzola cheese, and drizzle with the dressing mixture.

Ginger-Lime Chicken with Coconut Rice

Ingredients

- 1 ½ pounds skinless, boneless chicken breast halves - cut into 1 inch cubes

- 2 limes, zested and juiced

- 2 tablespoons grated fresh ginger root

- 1 ¾ cups coconut milk

- ½ teaspoon white sugar

- 1 cup jasmine rice

- 1 tablespoon sesame oil

- 1 tablespoon honey

- ¼ cup sweetened flaked coconut

How To Make

1. In a glass bowl, mix chicken breast cubes with lime juice, lime zest, and grated ginger. Let marinate for about 20 minutes.

2. In a medium saucepan, combine the coconut milk and sugar over medium-high heat. Bring to a simmer. Stir in the jasmine rice, reduce heat to low, and cook tightly covered for about 20 minutes or until liquid is absorbed. Remove from the heat and fluff rice with a fork; cover, and keep warm.

3. In a large skillet or wok, heat the sesame oil over medium-high heat. Add chicken and marinade. Stir fry until the chicken is nicely browned, about 3 minutes. Drizzle the honey onto the chicken and continue to stir-fry for another minute or so, being careful not to let the honey burn. Remove from the heat and sprinkle with coconut.

4. Serve hot with the coconut rice on the side.

Homemade Pickled Ginger (Gari)

Ingredients

- 8 ounces fresh young ginger root, peeled

- 1 ½ teaspoons sea salt

- 1 cup rice vinegar

- ⅓ cup white sugar

How To Make

1. Cut ginger into chunks. Place in a bowl, sprinkle with sea salt, and stir to coat. Let stand for about 30 minutes, then transfer to a clean lidded jar.

2. Stir together rice vinegar and sugar in a saucepan until sugar has dissolved. Bring to a boil, then pour the boiling liquid over ginger root pieces in the jar.

3. Allow the mixture to cool, then seal the jar. After a few minutes, the liquid may change to a slightly pinkish color; don't be alarmed. Store in the refrigerator for at least 1 week.

4. Cut pieces of ginger into paper-thin slices for serving.

CHAPTER 6
ALLERGIC RHINITIS-FRIENDLY
SOUP AND STEW

Citrus Wild Blueberry Sauce

Ingredients

- 2 cups frozen wild blueberries

- ½ cup orange juice

- 2 tablespoons fresh lemon juice

- 1 teaspoon lemon zest

- ¼ teaspoon ground cinnamon

- ¼ cup water

- 4 teaspoons cornstarch

- 2 tablespoons dark brown sugar

How To Make

1. Bring the blueberries, orange juice, and lemon juice to a boil in a small saucepan over medium heat. Stir in the lemon zest and cinnamon; adjust heat to low setting.

2. Whisk together the water and cornstarch until there are no lumps. Stir the cornstarch mixture and brown sugar into the blueberry mixture until thickened. Remove from heat and allow to rest for 10 minutes before using.

Carrot Ginger Creme

Ingredients

- 2 tablespoons canola oil

- 1 medium onion, chopped

- 2 pounds carrots, cut into medium dice

- 2 teaspoons ground ginger

- 4 cups vegetable broth

- 2 cups half-and-half

- salt and pepper to taste

How To Make

1. Heat oil in a large pot over medium heat. Cook and stir onion until translucent and tender, about

5 minutes. Stir in carrots, ginger, and vegetable broth, and simmer for 20 minutes, or until carrots are tender. Remove from heat and allow to cool slightly.

2. Transfer to a blender or food processor and blend until smooth. Return to soup pot, add half and half, and heat until warmed through. Season with salt and pepper, and serve.

Ginger Dipping Sauce

Ingredients

- ¼ cup chopped onion

- 1 clove garlic, minced

- 1 tablespoon minced fresh ginger root

- ½ lemon, juiced

- ¼ cup soy sauce

- ¼ teaspoon sugar

- ¼ teaspoon white vinegar

How To Make

1. In a blender, combine onion, garlic, ginger, lemon juice, soy sauce, sugar, and vinegar. Process until smooth. Serve at room temperature.

CHAPTER 7
PASTERY RECIPES FOR YOUR
TASTEBUDS

Citrus Egg Yolk Cookies

Ingredients

- 1 ½ cups white sugar

- 1 cup butter, softened

- 6 egg yolks

- 1 teaspoon vanilla extract

- ½ teaspoon lemon extract

- ½ teaspoon orange extract

- 2 ½ cups all-purpose flour

- 1 teaspoon baking soda

- 1 teaspoon cream of tartar

How To Make

1. Preheat oven to 350 degrees F (175 degrees C). Grease or line baking sheets with parchment paper.

2. Beat sugar and butter together in a bowl with an electric mixer until light and fluffy. Beat egg yolks, vanilla extract, lemon extract, and orange extract together in another bowl. Add egg yolk mixture to butter mixture; beat well.

3. Sift flour, baking soda, and cream of tartar together in a bowl. Stir flour mixture into butter mixture until dough is well-blended. Roll dough

into walnut-size balls and place on prepared baking sheets. Press dough balls to slightly flatten.

4. Bake in the preheated oven until golden around the edges and set, 8 to 10 minutes.

Citrus Cheesecake

Ingredients

• 1 egg yolk

• 1 tablespoon fresh lemon juice

• 1 teaspoon grated lemon zest

• ¼ teaspoon vanilla extract

• 1 ¼ cups all-purpose flour

- ⅓ cup white sugar

- ½ cup butter, room temperature

- 1 egg white

- 3 (8 ounce) packages cream cheese

- 1 ⅔ cups white sugar

- 2 tablespoons cornstarch

- 1 tablespoon fresh lemon juice

- 1 tablespoon grated orange zest

- 2 teaspoons grated lime zest

- 1 ½ teaspoons grated lemon zest

- ½ teaspoon vanilla extract

- 3 eggs

- 1 cup sour cream

- ⅔ cup orange marmalade

- 2 teaspoons fresh lemon juice

How To Make

1. Preheat oven to 450 degrees F (230 degrees C). Butter a 9 inch springform pan. In a small bowl, whisk together egg yolk, 1 tablespoon lemon juice, 1 teaspoon lemon peel and 1/4 teaspoon vanilla. In the bowl of a food processor, combine flour and 1/3 cup sugar. Add butter and process until coarse crumbs form. With machine running, add yolk mixture and blend until moist clumps form. Press dough onto bottom and 1 1/2 inches up sides of prepared pan. Freeze crust 10 minutes.

2. Brush crust lightly with egg white. Bake until crust is pale golden, about 15 minutes. Cool on

rack while preparing filling. Reduce oven temperature to 350 degrees F (175 degrees C).

3. In a large bowl, beat cream cheese and 1 2/3 cups sugar until smooth. Beat in cornstarch, 1 tablespoon lemon juice, orange zest, lime zest, 1 1/2 teaspoon lemon zest and 1/2 teaspoon vanilla. Beat in eggs one at a time, then stir in sour cream. Pour filling into crust.

4. Bake in the preheated oven for 55 to 60 minutes, or until puffed and cracked around edges and center moves only slightly when pan is gently shaken. Allow to cool to room temperature, then refrigerate overnight.

5. In a saucepan over medium heat, boil marmalade and 2 teaspoons lemon juice until slightly reduced, about 2 minutes. Spread warm glaze on top of cake. Chill cake 10 minutes.

Remove pan sides and transfer cake to serving plate.

Citrus Shortbread Cookies

Ingredients

- 2 cups all-purpose flour

- ¼ teaspoon baking powder

- ⅛ teaspoon salt

- 1 cup butter, softened

- ¾ cup confectioners' sugar

- 2 teaspoons vanilla extract

- ½ teaspoon almond extract

- 1 tablespoon grated orange zest, or more to taste

- 2 cups sweetened dried cranberries, chopped

How To Make

1. Combine flour, baking powder, and salt in a bowl; set aside. Beat the butter and confectioners' sugar with an electric mixer in a large bowl until smooth. Stir in the vanilla and almond extracts and orange zest. Mix in the flour mixture until just incorporated. Fold in the cranberries; mixing just enough to evenly combine.

2. Divide the dough into 2 equal portions, then roll into logs about 7 inches long. Wrap each log in wax paper or plastic wrap, and chill in the refrigerator for at least 4 hours.

3. Preheat an oven to 350 degrees F (175 degrees C).

4. Remove wax paper, and cut the cookie dough into 1/2-inch slices. Arrange the slices on a baking sheet about 1 inch apart.

5. Bake in the preheated oven until firm but not browned, about 10 minutes.

Rainbow Citrus Cake

Ingredients

- 3 ½ cups all-purpose flour

- 5 teaspoons baking powder

- 1 teaspoon salt

- ¾ cup shortening

- 2 ¼ cups white sugar

* 4 eggs, room temperature

* 1 ½ cups milk

* 2 teaspoons vanilla extract

* 2 teaspoons grated lemon zest

* 2 teaspoons grated orange zest

* 2 teaspoons grated lime zest

* 2 drops yellow food coloring

* 2 drops orange food coloring

* 2 drops green food coloring

* 1 recipe Lemon Custard Filling

* 1 recipe Orange Cream Frosting

Ingredients

1. Preheat oven to 350 degrees F (175 degrees C). Grease and flour three 9-inch pans. Sift together the flour, baking powder, and salt. Set aside.

2. In a large bowl, cream together the shortening and sugar until light and fluffy. Beat in the eggs one at a time, mixing until each egg is incorporated; stir in the vanilla. Beat in the flour mixture alternately with the milk. Divide batter into 3 bowls.

3. In the first bowl, stir in lemon zest and yellow food coloring; pour into prepared pan. In the second bowl, stir in orange zest and orange food coloring; pour into second prepared pan. In the last bowl, stir in the lime zest and green food coloring; pour into third prepared pan.

4. Bake in the preheated oven until a toothpick inserted into the center of each cake layer comes

out clean, about 30 minutes. Let cool in pan for 5 minutes, then turn out onto a wire rack and cool completely.

5. Assemble the cake: stack the layers together with the Lemon Filling in between the layers. Frost sides and top with Orange Cream Frosting. Refrigerate until serving.

Ginger Bars

Ingredients

- 1 ¾ cups brown sugar

- ⅔ cup butter

- ¼ cup molasses

- 2 teaspoons ground ginger

- 2 eggs

- 2 teaspoons vanilla extract

- 1 cup all-purpose flour

- 1 cup whole wheat flour

- 1 teaspoon baking powder

- ¼ teaspoon baking soda

- 1 teaspoon salt

Ingredients

1. Preheat oven to 350 degrees F (175 degrees C). Grease a 9x13-inch baking pan.

2. Mash the brown sugar, butter, and molasses together in a bowl with a spoon until the mixture

is creamy and thoroughly combined. Mix in the ginger, eggs, and vanilla extract. In a separate bowl, combine the all-purpose flour, whole wheat flour, baking powder, baking soda, and salt. Stir 1/4 of flour mixture into the butter mixture at a time, incorporating each addition before adding the next. Pour the batter into the prepared baking pan.

3. Bake in the preheated oven until a toothpick inserted into the center comes out clean, 25 to 30 minutes. Let cool before cutting.

Triple the Ginger Cookies

Ingredients

- ¾ cup butter

- 1 cup packed brown sugar

- 1 egg

- ¼ cup molasses

- 2 ¼ cups all-purpose flour

- 2 teaspoons ground ginger

- 2 teaspoons baking soda

- ½ teaspoon salt

- 1 ½ tablespoons minced fresh ginger root

- ½ cup chopped crystallized ginger

How To Make

1. In a large bowl, cream together the butter and brown sugar until smooth. Beat in the egg and molasses. Combine the flour, ground ginger,

baking soda, and salt; stir into the molasses mixture using a wooden spoon. Mix in the fresh and crystallized gingers. Cover, and refrigerate dough for at least 2 hours, or overnight.

2. Preheat oven to 350 degrees F (175 degrees C). Shape dough into 1 inch balls, and place about 2 inches apart onto ungreased cookie sheet.

3. Bake for 10 minutes in the preheated oven, or until lightly browned. Cool on wire racks.

Chewy Ginger Cookies

Ingredients

• 2 cups sifted all-purpose flour

• 4 teaspoons ground ginger

- 2 teaspoons baking soda

- 2 teaspoons ground cinnamon

- ½ teaspoon salt

- ¼ teaspoon ground allspice

- 1 cup white sugar

- ¾ cup butter, softened

- 1 egg

- ¼ cup dark molasses

- ⅓ cup chopped crystallized ginger (Optional)

How To Make

1. Preheat oven to 350 degrees F (175 degrees C).

2. Sift the flour, ground ginger, baking soda, cinnamon, salt, and allspice together into a mixing bowl; stir.

3. Beat sugar and butter with an electric mixer in a large bowl until smooth and creamy. Beat egg and molasses into creamed butter mixture. Gradually stir flour mixture into butter mixture until just coming together into a batter. Gently fold crystallized ginger through the batter.

4. Roll rounded teaspoon-sized amounts of dough into small balls between your hands and place onto ungreased baking sheets about 2 inches apart.

5. Bake in preheated oven until the tops are rounded and slightly cracked, about 10 minutes. Cool cookies on baking sheets for 1 minute before removing to a wire rack to cool completely.

Mom's Ginger Snaps

Ingredients

- 1 cup packed brown sugar

- ¾ cup vegetable oil

- ¼ cup molasses

- 1 large egg

- 2 cups all-purpose flour

- 2 teaspoons baking soda

- 1 teaspoon ground ginger

- 1 teaspoon ground cinnamon

- ½ teaspoon ground cloves

- ¼ teaspoon salt

- ⅓ cup white sugar for decoration

How To Make

1. Preheat the oven to 375 degrees F (190 degrees C).

2. Mix together brown sugar, oil, molasses, and egg in a large bowl.

3. Combine flour, baking soda, ginger, cinnamon, cloves, and salt; stir into the molasses mixture.

4. Roll dough into 1 1/4-inch balls. Roll each ball in white sugar before placing 2 inches apart on ungreased cookie sheets.

5. Bake for 10 to 12 minutes in the preheated oven, or until center is firm. Cool on wire racks.

Boscobel Beach Ginger Cake

Ingredients

- 2 ½ cups all-purpose flour

- 4 teaspoons baking powder

- 4 teaspoons ground ginger

- 1 ½ teaspoons ground cinnamon

- ½ teaspoon salt

- 1 cup butter

- 1 ¼ cups packed brown sugar

- 4 eggs

- ¼ cup grated fresh ginger root

- 1 teaspoon vanilla extract

- 1 cup milk

- 2 tablespoons confectioners' sugar for dusting

How To Make

1. Preheat the oven to 350 degrees F (175 degrees C). Grease and flour a 9-inch fluted tube pan, such as Bundt.

2. Sift together flour, baking powder, ground ginger, cinnamon, and salt. Set aside.

3. In a large bowl, cream together butter and brown sugar until light and fluffy. Beat in eggs one at a time, then stir in grated ginger root and vanilla. Beat in flour mixture alternately with milk,

mixing just until incorporated. Pour batter into the prepared pan.

4. Bake in the preheated oven for 45 to 50 minutes, or until a toothpick inserted into the center of the cake comes out clean. Let cool in pan for 10 minutes, then turn out onto a serving plate. Dust lightly with confectioners' sugar before serving.

Ginger Crinkles

Ingredients

- ⅔ cup vegetable oil

- 1 cup white sugar

- 1 egg

- ¼ cup molasses

- 2 cups all-purpose flour

- 2 teaspoons baking soda

- 1 teaspoon ground cinnamon

- 1 teaspoon ground ginger

- ¼ cup white sugar

- ½ teaspoon salt

How To Make

1. Mix oil and sugar thoroughly with electric mixer. Add egg and mix well. Pour in molasses. Sift and add dry *Ingredients* until incorporated.

2. Roll teaspoonful of dough into ball, drop into sugar to coat.

3. Place on ungreased cookie sheet. Bake at 350 degrees F (175 degrees C) for 15 minutes.

Fresh Ginger Cookies

Ingredients

- 2 ¼ cups all-purpose flour

- 1 teaspoon baking soda

- ½ teaspoon salt

- 1 ¼ cups white sugar, divided, or more to taste

- ¾ cup unsalted butter, softened

- 2 tablespoons grated fresh ginger

- ¼ cup molasses

• 1 large egg

How To Make

1. Combine flour, baking soda, and salt in a large bowl.

2. Beat 1 cup sugar, butter, and ginger in a large bowl with an electric mixer until light and fluffy. Beat in molasses and egg. Gently fold in flour mixture until just combined. Chill for 1 hour.

3. Preheat the oven to 350 degrees F (175 degrees C).

4. Roll chilled dough into 1 1/2 inch balls. Roll balls in remaining sugar, then place 2 inches apart onto ungreased baking sheets.

5. Bake in the preheated oven until mostly (but not fully) set in the centers and edges are starting to

brown, about 15 minutes. Let stand for 1 minute on the baking sheets, then remove to wire racks and let cool completely.

Whole Wheat Ginger Snaps

Ingredients

• 1 cup butter or margarine

• 1 ½ cups white sugar

• 2 eggs, beaten

• 1 cup molasses

• 4 cups whole wheat flour

• 1 tablespoon baking soda

* 2 teaspoons baking powder

* 1 tablespoon ground ginger

* 1 ½ teaspoons ground nutmeg

* 1 ½ teaspoons ground cinnamon

* 1 ½ teaspoons ground cloves

* 1 ½ teaspoons ground allspice

* 1 cup white sugar for decoration

How To Make

1. Preheat the oven to 350 degrees F (175 degrees C). Grease cookie sheets.

2. In a large bowl, cream together the butter and 1 1/2 cups of sugar until smooth. Mix in the eggs, and then the molasses. Combine the whole wheat

flour, baking soda, baking powder, ginger, nutmeg, cinnamon, cloves, and allspice, heaping the measures if you like a lot of spice. Stir the dry ingredients into the molasses mixture just until blended.

3. Roll the dough into small balls, and dip the top of each ball into the remaining white sugar. Place the cookies about 2 inches apart on the cookie sheets.

4. Bake for 10 to 15 minutes in the preheated oven, until the tops are cracked. Bake longer for crispy cookies, less time for chewy cookies. Cool on wire racks.

Ginger Pear Bread

Ingredients

- 1 cup peeled, cored, and chopped pears

- ½ cup white sugar

- ½ teaspoon ground ginger

- ¼ teaspoon ground cloves

- 1 cup all-purpose flour

- 1 teaspoon baking soda

- ½ teaspoon salt

- ¼ teaspoon baking powder

- ⅓ cup vegetable oil

- 2 large eggs, beaten

- 1 teaspoon vanilla extract

How To Make

1. Toss chopped pears with sugar, ginger, and cloves in a large bowl. Set aside until sugar dissolves, 10 to 15 minutes.

2. Preheat the oven to 325 degrees F (165 degrees C). Grease an 8x4-inch loaf pan.

3. Combine flour, baking soda, salt, and baking powder in a bowl.

4. Stir oil, eggs, and vanilla into pears. Add flour mixture and gently stir until just combined. Pour into the prepared loaf pan.

5. Bake in the preheated oven until golden brown and a toothpick inserted in the center comes out clean, about 40 minutes.

FROGHOPPER's Candied Ginger Carrots

Ingredients

• 1 (12 ounce) package baby carrots

• 1 cup water

• 3 tablespoons butter

• 2 tablespoons brown sugar

• 1 ½ teaspoons ground ginger

• ¼ teaspoon salt

How To Make

1. Bring carrots and water to a boil in a saucepan, reduce heat to low, and simmer until the carrots are tender, about 10 minutes. Drain carrots; stir in butter until carrots are coated. Stir in brown sugar, ginger, and salt; bring to a boil, and cook the carrots, stirring often, until the carrots are glazed, 2 to 3 minutes.

Ginger Banana Bread

Ingredients

• 2 cups all-purpose flour

• 1 teaspoon baking soda

• 1 teaspoon ground cinnamon

• ¼ teaspoon ground nutmeg

- ¼ teaspoon ground ginger

- ¼ teaspoon salt

- ½ cup butter, softened

- ½ cup white sugar

- ½ cup brown sugar

- 2 ⅓ cups mashed overripe bananas

- 2 eggs, beaten

- 1 tablespoon lemon juice

- 1 teaspoon vanilla extract

How To Make

1. Preheat oven to 350 degrees F (175 degrees C). Lightly grease a 9x5-inch loaf pan.

2. Combine flour, baking soda, cinnamon, nutmeg, ginger, and salt together in a bowl.

3. Beat butter, white sugar, and brown sugar together in a bowl using an electric mixer until smooth and creamy. Stir bananas, eggs, lemon juice, and vanilla extract into creamed butter mixture until well blended. Stir banana mixture into flour mixture until batter is just combined; pour into the prepared pan.

4. Bake in the preheated oven until a toothpick inserted in the center of the loaf comes out clean, 60 to 65 minutes. Cool bread in the pan for 10 minutes before turning onto a wire rack to cool completely.

Notes:

If you want to bake in a smaller pan, then shorten the baking time to 40 or 45 minutes. If you are using decorative wooden lattice bread pans (common during the holidays for gift-giving) remember to increase the temperature by 25 degrees.

Pumpkin Ginger Cupcakes

Ingredients

• 2 cups all-purpose flour

• 1 (3.4 ounce) package instant butterscotch pudding mix

• ⅓ cup finely chopped crystallized ginger

• 1 tablespoon ground cinnamon

• 2 teaspoons baking soda

- ½ teaspoon ground ginger

- ½ teaspoon ground allspice

- ¼ teaspoon ground cloves

- ¼ teaspoon salt

- 1 cup butter, room temperature

- 1 cup white sugar

- 1 cup packed brown sugar

- 4 large eggs, room temperature

- 1 (15 ounce) can pumpkin puree

- 1 teaspoon vanilla extract

How To Make

1. Preheat the oven to 350 degrees F (175 degrees C). Grease 24 muffin cups or line with paper liners.

2. Whisk together flour, pudding mix, crystallized ginger, cinnamon, baking soda, ground ginger, allspice, cloves, and salt in a bowl; set aside.

3. Beat butter, white sugar, and brown sugar in a large bowl with an electric mixer until light and fluffy. Add eggs one at a time, mixing well after each addition; beat in pumpkin purée and vanilla with last egg. Stir in flour mixture, mixing until just combined. Divide batter between the prepared muffin cups.

4. Bake in the preheated oven until golden and the tops spring back when lightly pressed, about 20 minutes. Cool muffins in the pans for 10 minutes before removing to cool completely on a wire rack.

Big Soft Ginger Cookies

Ingredients

- 2 tablespoons white sugar

- 2 ¼ cups all-purpose flour

- 2 teaspoons ground ginger

- 1 teaspoon baking soda

- ¾ teaspoon ground cinnamon

- ½ teaspoon ground cloves

- ¼ teaspoon salt

- ¾ cup margarine, softened

- 1 cup white sugar

- 1 large egg

- ¼ cup molasses

- 1 tablespoon water

How To Make

1. Preheat the oven to 350 degrees F (175 degrees C). Set 2 tablespoons sugar in a small bowl; set aside.

2. Sift together flour, ginger, baking soda, cinnamon, cloves, and salt in a bowl.

3. Cream margarine and remaining 1 cup sugar in a large bowl until light and fluffy. Beat in egg, then stir in molasses and water. Gradually stir the sifted ingredients into the molasses mixture until well combined.

4. Use floured hands to shape dough into 24 walnut-sized balls. Roll each ball in the reserved sugar until coated. Place cookies 2 inches apart onto ungreased cookie sheets, and flatten slightly with the bottom of a glass.

5. Bake in the preheated oven for 8 to 10 minutes, switching racks halfway through.

6. Remove from the oven and allow cookies to cool on the baking sheets for 5 minutes, then transfer to a wire rack to cool completely.

Papaya Surprise Smoothie

Ingredients

- 1 papaya - peeled, seeded and diced

- 1 banana, peeled and sliced

- ½ cup sliced fresh strawberries

- ⅓ cup milk

- ¼ cup sugar

- 15 ice cubes

How To Make

1. In a blender, blend the papaya, banana, strawberries, milk, sugar, and ice cubes until smooth.

Papaya Passion Smoothie

Ingredients

• 2 cups papaya - peeled, seeded and cubed

• 2 cups milk

• ¼ cup white sugar

• ¼ cup sweetened condensed milk

• 1 cup vanilla yogurt

- 2 tablespoons cream cheese

- 2 cups ice

How To Make

1. Place papaya, milk, sugar, condensed milk, yogurt, cream cheese, and ice in a blender. Blend until smooth. Serve immediately.

Tropical Fruit Smoothie

Ingredients

- 1 mango, peeled and seeded

- 1 papaya, peeled and seeded

- ½ cup fresh strawberries

- ⅓ cup orange juice

- 5 cubes ice

How To Make

1. Combine mango, papaya, strawberries, orange juice, and ice cubes in a blender; blend until smooth.

Supercharged Smoothie

Ingredients

- 1 cup almond milk

- ½ cup fresh papaya

- 1 scoop protein powder

- 1 (1 inch) piece peeled and chopped fresh turmeric root

- 1 (1/2 inch) piece fresh ginger root, peeled

- 3 cubes ice, or as desired

How To Make

1. Combine almond milk, papaya, protein powder, turmeric root, and ginger root in a blender; add ice and blend until smooth.

Ginger Berry Smoothie

Ingredients

- 1 cup water, or more as needed

- ¼ cup frozen blueberries

• 4 frozen strawberries, or more to taste

• 1 (1 inch) piece fresh ginger, peeled and coarsely chopped

• 1 tablespoon agave nectar

Ingredients

1. Blend water, blueberries, strawberries, ginger, and agave nectar together in a blender until thick and smooth.

Ginger Fruit Smoothie

Ingredients

• 1 cup water, or more as needed

• ¼ cup frozen blueberries

- ¼ cup seedless green grapes

- ½ green apple, cored and chopped

- 3 frozen strawberries, or more to taste

- 1 (1 inch) piece peeled fresh ginger, cut into thirds

- 1 tablespoon agave nectar

How To Make

1. Blend water, blueberries, grapes, apple, strawberries, ginger, and agave nectar together in a blender until thick and slushy.

Green Smoothie with Ginger

Ingredients

- 2 cups fresh spinach leaves, or to taste

- 1 cup water, or as needed

- 1 medium apple, cored and chopped

- 1 medium pear, cored and chopped

- 1 small lemon, juiced

- 2 tablespoons flaxseed meal

- ½ teaspoon freshly grated ginger

How To Make

1. Combine spinach, 1 cup water, apple, pear, lemon juice, flaxseed, and ginger in a blender. Puree until smooth, adding more water if needed.

Note:

Add fresh fruit, cucumbers, slivered almonds, coconut, fresh herbs, or different dark leafy greens for tasty variations on this recipe.

Citrus Healthy Smoothie

Ingredients

- 2 frozen bananas, cut into small chunks

- 2 cups frozen pineapple chunks

- 1 cup fresh orange juice

- 1 cup coconut milk

- 1 lime, juiced

- 2 teaspoons ground turmeric

- 1 (1/2 inch) piece fresh ginger, peeled and chopped

- ½ teaspoon ground nutmeg

- ice cubes as desired

How To Make

1. Blend bananas, pineapple, orange juice, coconut milk, lime juice, turmeric, ginger, nutmeg, and ice cubes together in a blender until smooth.

CHAPTER 9
WHAT ARE YOUR TREATMENT CHOICES?

The approach to treating rhinitis hinges on identifying and addressing its underlying cause or diagnosis. In cases where a specific trigger can be identified and avoided, this preventative measure can serve as a beneficial therapy. For instance, individuals with cat allergies may experience symptom reduction by avoiding cat exposure and direct contact with cats.

Medications play a crucial role in managing rhinitis symptoms. Depending on the precise source of the symptoms, various drugs may be prescribed, including saline spray or rinse for nasal irrigation, oral or intranasal antihistamines to alleviate allergy symptoms, corticosteroids typically administered as an intranasal spray to reduce nasal inflammation, and intranasal spray of ipratropium bromide to alleviate nasal congestion.

Allergen immunotherapy represents another treatment option for allergic rhinitis. This therapy, often administered in the form of allergy injections, pills, or liquid drops placed under the tongue, aims to desensitize individuals to specific allergens over time. However, the suitability of allergen immunotherapy as a treatment option should be evaluated by a skilled ear, nose, and throat (ENT) physician or allergist based on individual circumstances.

In cases where medications fail to provide adequate relief for severe runny nose or nasal obstruction/congestion, further office-based treatments or surgical interventions may be recommended by your ENT specialist. These interventions aim to address underlying anatomical issues contributing to nasal symptoms and may include procedures such as nasal septoplasty or turbinate reduction.

What Queries Should I Pose to My Physician?

- - What might be the leading cause behind the manifestation of my rhinitis symptoms, and could there be multiple factors contributing to its onset?

- - Considering the complexity of my symptoms, would undergoing allergy testing be a beneficial step to comprehensively identify and understand the specific triggers exacerbating my condition?

- - In addition to identifying triggers through testing, could adopting a proactive approach by avoiding certain allergens or environmental factors contribute significantly to symptom relief and overall improvement in my quality of life?

- - Given the diverse range of medications available, which ones would be the most suitable and effective in managing my rhinitis symptoms, considering factors such as severity, frequency, and individual responsiveness?

- - Furthermore, are there any additional diagnostic assessments required to gain a comprehensive understanding of my condition? Would conducting specific laboratory tests provide valuable insights into underlying factors contributing to my symptoms? Additionally, would seeking consultations with other medical specialists offer further expertise and perspectives in devising an optimal treatment plan tailored to my unique needs and circumstances?

Your personalized treatment regimen may consist of the subsequent elements.

- • Implementing changes in lifestyle, such as environmental control measures, represents a pivotal aspect of managing allergic rhinitis, aiming to minimize exposure to allergens and mitigate symptoms.

• • Incorporating medication targeted specifically for the nasal passages serves to alleviate inflammation, providing relief from the discomfort associated with allergic rhinitis.

• • Antihistamines play a crucial role in reducing itching, sneezing, and a runny nose, effectively addressing the hallmark symptoms of allergic rhinitis and enhancing overall comfort.

• • Decongestants serve as another pharmacological option to relieve nasal congestion, facilitating improved breathing and nasal airflow for individuals grappling with allergic rhinitis.

* • Alongside the aforementioned medications, other drugs or immunotherapy treatments may be considered, provided they align with the individual's specific medical needs and circumstances, offering a comprehensive approach to managing allergic rhinitis tailored to each patient's requirements and preferences.

* By embracing a multifaceted treatment approach encompassing lifestyle modifications, targeted medication, and potentially immunotherapy, individuals can effectively manage allergic rhinitis and experience improved quality of life despite the challenges posed by this condition. It is essential to consult healthcare professionals to determine the most suitable treatment

regimen tailored to individual needs and preferences, ensuring optimal management and symptom relief.

How about allergy injections?

Allergy injections, while not suitable for everyone, should not instill fear. Many patients have reported significant improvements in their allergy symptoms by following their treatment plans, which often include lifestyle modifications and prescribed medications. If allergen immunotherapy, commonly known as allergy injections, is deemed appropriate for your condition, your doctor will gladly address any concerns or inquiries you may have regarding the treatment process.

Typically, patients undergoing allergen immunotherapy receive injections once or twice a week initially, followed by a transition to once-a-month injections over the course of several years. This gradual schedule allows the body to build tolerance to specific allergens, ultimately reducing the severity of allergic reactions.

It's essential to recognize that the decision to pursue allergen immunotherapy should be made in consultation with a healthcare professional who can assess your individual health needs and tailor a treatment plan accordingly. Your doctor will evaluate various factors, including the severity of your allergies, your medical history, and your lifestyle, to determine if allergy injections are the most suitable option for managing your condition.

Furthermore, understanding the process and benefits of allergen immunotherapy can alleviate any apprehensions you may have. By gradually exposing your immune system to allergens through controlled injections, the body learns to tolerate these substances, reducing the frequency and severity of allergic reactions over time. This approach not only provides relief from bothersome symptoms but also addresses the underlying cause of allergies, offering long-term benefits for overall health and well-being.

In addition to allergen immunotherapy, your treatment plan may include other interventions to manage allergy symptoms effectively. These may encompass lifestyle modifications such as minimizing exposure to allergens, implementing dietary changes, and incorporating over-the-counter or prescription medications as needed.

Remember, effective management of allergies often requires a comprehensive approach that addresses both symptom relief and underlying immune system sensitivities. By working closely with your healthcare provider and adhering to your personalized treatment plan, you can take proactive steps towards improving your quality of life and enjoying greater freedom from allergy-related discomfort.